# The Acid Reflux Solution

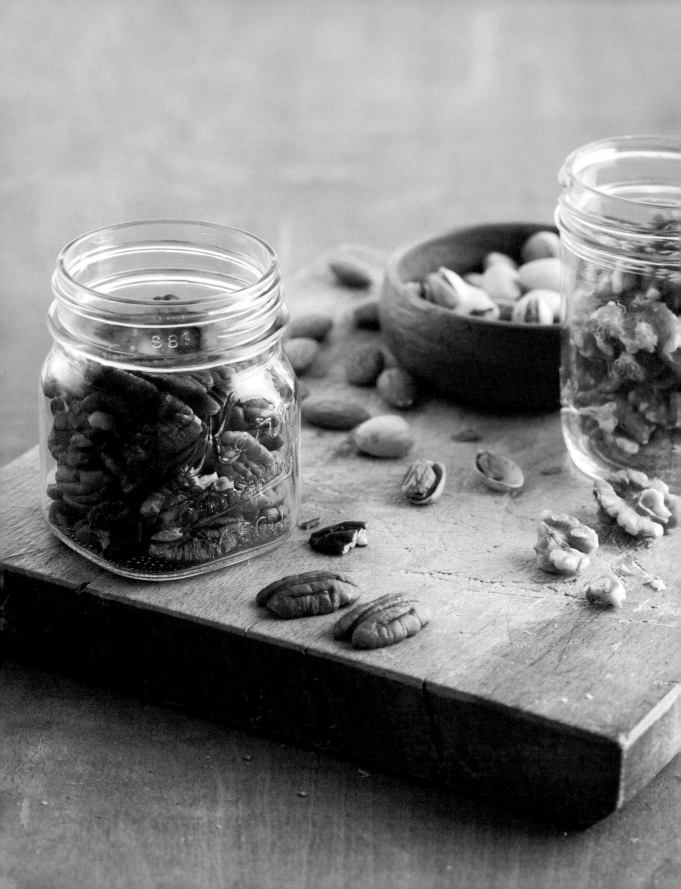

# THE
# ACID REFLUX SOLUTION

### A COOKBOOK AND LIFESTYLE GUIDE FOR
## Healing Heartburn Naturally

## Jorge E. Rodriguez, MD

with SUSAN WYLER, MPH, RD

*Photography by Jennifer Martiné*

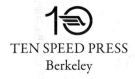

TEN SPEED PRESS
Berkeley

This book is dedicated to my parents, Ofelia and
Juan, who sacrificed it all for their children . . .
and to Whoopi and especially Tom, for believing,
believing, and then believing some more.

# CONTENTS

8/20/12 Ingram

# ACKNOWLEDGMENTS

**WE WOULD LIKE TO THANK** our intrepid editor, Julie Bennett, whose attention to detail and dedication to quality made this a better book than it would have been without her. We also appreciate the efforts of designer Katy Brown, copy editor Leslie Evans, proofreader Karen Levy, and photographer Jennifer Martiné for their excellent work.

Jorge would like to thank Susan Wyler for her endless dedication to this work and for her tireless friendship, Carole Bidnick for her sage guidance, and last but not least, Nancy Udell and MaryAnn Palumbo for getting this ball rolling.

Susan wishes to thank Dr. Jorge, whose boundless energy, medical integrity, and generous good nature made this collaboration such a delight, and agent Carole Bidnick, for making such a happy match. She would like to acknowledge the databases and helpfulness of the librarians at the health sciences library at the University of North Carolina at Chapel Hill, which greatly facilitated the research for this book. And thanks especially to her professor and advisor, the exceptional Amanda S. Holliday, MS, RD, LDN, who served as teacher, mentor, and role model.

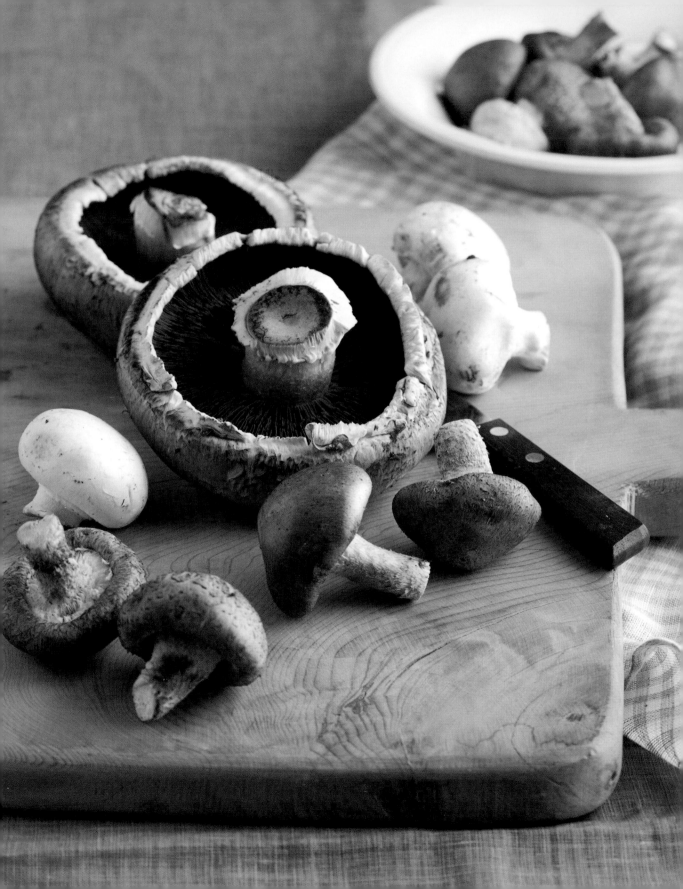

# INTRODUCTION

*I Feel Your Pain*

BLUE CHEESE BURGERS, SPAGHETTI AND MEATBALLS, Spanish chicken and rice . . . these are just a few of my favorite dishes that I could not enjoy without paying a high price until I developed the Acid Reflux Solution. Growing up in South Florida, Southern California, and the Detroit area gave me a broad appreciation of American culinary culture as it came into its own in the '80s and '90s. Growing up Cuban in those places offered me some of the tastiest cooking on earth wherever I was.

My mother's Cuban cooking, although delicious, could have caused acid reflux in a giraffe. And it certainly was not geared to weight control. All that braised pork cooked in lard with *mojo de ajo*—an intense garlic and lemon sauce—and black beans and rice in portions that made supersize look wimpy guaranteed that as I developed physically, so did my girth, and by the time I was a practicing physician, my weight could be classified as obese (even though I didn't look that heavy). At the same time, until this past year, I've suffered from GERD, or gastroesophageal reflux disease, my entire adult life. Think there might have been a connection? Somehow, it never occurred to me. Why should it? For me, heartburn was simply what happened whenever you ate. I didn't need an alarm clock to wake up. All the garlic, onions, and lemon did it for me—usually about an hour after I went to bed following a substantial late supper or midnight snack, with the pain of heartburn unmistakable as the searing acid escaped my stomach and shot up my throat.

Heartburn, the chief complaint of GERD, is one of the most prevalent medical problems in America, with roughly a sixth of the population reporting symptoms at least once a week. Expenditures for powerful antacids like proton pump inhibitors total seven billion dollars a year, making Nexium the second most popular drug in the country. Yet too little attention is given to what is ultimately the most effective and natural long-term solution to acid reflux: a sensible combination of healthy eating and lifestyle modifications that include regular physical activity.

Does the prescription of diet and exercise sound familiar? It should, because obesity and GERD are inextricably linked, with a prevalence two to three times that of people with normal weight status. If I sound passionate about this problem it's because I have a double interest: As an expert in gastroenterology, I've treated tens of thousands of patients suffering from acid reflux and performed thousands of endoscopies to confirm my diagnosis or perform corrective procedures. Why I was drawn to this area of medicine I'm not entirely sure, but even as an impressionable young medical student, the intimate association with the inside of the body fascinated me. The first time I watched an endoscopy, a high-tech fiber-optic internal examination of the esophagus and stomach, I was mesmerized. I remember thinking: "How extraordinary! It feels like you are actually walking through the inside of the body." Internal medicine had me hooked from then on.

For a long time, I did a lot of thinking about my patients and not much about myself. I didn't worry about my weight, or my GERD; both were simply facts of life. I believed that in the future I could deal with both when it became impossible to ignore them any longer. But the clock kept ticking as I became accustomed to living with obesity and GERD. I treated my own illness the same way I treated my patients—with over-the-counter antacids and prescription medications. In the back of my mind, I remembered the fact sheets that came with the drugs, suggesting use for no longer than four to six weeks, but what can you do when your heartburn persists?

It was almost by accident that I connected the dots and figured out what to do—for myself and for my patients. The approach to healing by combining medical expertise with lifestyle changes had been building for a long time.

## A Better Way

I've been a dedicated practicing physician since 1983. Medicine is my calling and my passion. Slowly over time, as I got to know my patients better, I began to see that illness and healing were a lot more than I'd been taught in medical school. A great deal of conscientious medicine is not just writing prescription drugs and performing surgical procedures. It involves understanding the individual patient in his or her totality as a person. I realized that to be a truly fine doctor, I had to look beyond my expert knowledge base, to have a dialogue with my patients, so that besides analyzing their immediate physical symptoms, which were of course of prime importance, I also had to consider their diet, nutrition, physical activity, and spiritual or emotional well-being.

Instinctively, I knew I needed to find a better way. I wanted the antacid prescriptions to serve their proper purpose: as a tool for keeping heartburn under control while people took time to adjust their eating habits and behavior so that acid reflux was reduced naturally. I began recommending lifestyle changes to my patients diagnosed with GERD, suggesting ways that would alleviate their symptoms gradually and naturally, so I could wean them off the long-term use of pills. Some ideas, such as raising the head of the bed to prevent reflux, are standard medical procedure for preventing aspiration when hospital patients eat in bed. I applied others, such as appropriate portion sizes and food combinations from the research I conducted. I made further changes to my plan when I saw how patients responded to different recipes. But it wasn't until I organized all of my thoughts for this book that I put everything together. Only then did I make the connection between what I was preaching and what I was doing in terms of my own weight and my own health. You could say my eureka moment came on the end of a fork.

## An Evidence-Based Solution

It was my agent who introduced me to Susan Wyler, a cookbook writer and food editor who had gone back to school to study nutrition at the University of North Carolina at Chapel Hill. Though I'm a passable home cook, I am nowhere near equipped to develop my own recipes. I was looking for a food professional who would be comfortable with scientific literature, someone who could collaborate with me to condense what I had learned from working with my patients and what was scientifically proven about diet and acid reflux. I wanted a collection of recipes that would encompass a way of eating in terms of high fiber, low saturated fat, and portion control rather than a formulaic diet. Most of all, I wanted food that was delicious, easy to make, and satisfying—no deprivation required. Tossing old-fashioned myths about acid reflux out the window helped us a lot.

Susan agreed with me completely. Having recently studied GERD in her medical nutrition therapy class, she wanted all the recipes in this book to be what is called "evidence based." What does that mean? Simply that the information given is based on scientific evidence rather than someone's opinion or a way that has been followed traditionally because it "seems" to be effective. You might think all medical advice is evidence based, but unfortunately, sometimes people do things just because they've always been done that way. It's tradition, in other words. Sometimes it looks as if one thing causes another, but that is not necessarily the case. Just because two events occur together does not always mean they are related.

As an example, for years stomach ulcers were a major medical problem that medications were only partially successful in treating. People sometimes died from bleeding ulcers. To quell symptoms and supposedly help cure the problem, doctors and dieticians put patients on what was called the "sippy diet." It consisted of thick, creamy liquids like milk shakes, heavy cream, and cream soups, which would supposedly "coat" the stomach and prevent acid erosion. There was absolutely no scientific proof this worked, but it was standard medical practice. For many years, every doctor prescribed the sippy diet to their ulcer patients—until a brilliant, eccentric researcher proved that bacteria could indeed thrive even within the very low pH of the stomach, which no one would believe until he infected himself with *Heliobacter pylori* and promptly developed a painful duodenal ulcer. Most ulcers had nothing to do with diet and a lot to do with a bacterial infection.

So we've learned that just because something has been accepted as standard procedure does not always mean it's true. Evidence-based practice means you keep up with the very latest studies and experiments, evaluate them for the quality of the work, and then incorporate this new knowledge into your treatment plan for individuals you think will benefit. So Susan and I put our heads together to figure out what would be the best nutrition plan for alleviating or at least minimizing attacks of GERD.

# Creating the Acid Reflux Solution

We scoured the scientific literature to search for which foods physically triggered reflux—not just in anecdotal reports. To our surprise, there were fewer than a dozen, which we'll discuss in detail in chapter 4. Then we put our heads together with what we knew about digestion in general and medical nutrition therapy for GERD and other digestive problems—and combined that information with the success I'd been having in my practice—to decide what kind of diet would help the most in alleviating heartburn, bloating, and feeling stuffed and uncomfortable. We also drew from my extensive list of easy but effective lifestyle changes that can affect digestion in general and acid reflux in particular.

Next came my posing as a guinea pig. If I was going to recommend certain recipes to my readers, I wanted to make sure they worked. So I tried them first, because no one I knew was more susceptible to acid reflux than I was. I particularly requested a few recipes that reminded me of my childhood and Cuban heritage. How could I put my name on a book that didn't include some version of arroz con pollo (Spanish chicken with rice) or Cuban black bean soup? Before I handed Susan's recipes off to my patients, I tried them myself. From the first bite, it became clear that this food was so tasty and satisfying that it would become my standard fare. And it was then that I began to lose weight.

At the same time, and sooner than I expected, I started feeling a little better. Those really severe, unexpected attacks of acid reflux in the middle of the night were fewer and farther apart. All my patients who tried the recipes and complied with our lifestyle recommendations, especially including not drinking alcohol and sticking to portion control, did not have any reflux after their meals, either. Only after we developed the Acid Reflux Solution—our "recipe" for a reflux-free diet—did we realize that with no intention of designing a weight-loss plan, it had happened. Because if you follow the "rules" for reflux-free eating, especially portion control, you will naturally lose weight without even thinking about it. How great is that?

In the coming chapters, I'm going to talk about what acid reflux is, so you understand exactly what's happening in your body to cause your painful symptoms, and why GERD has become such an epidemic. We'll review all the medications prescribed for heartburn, including what's good about them and how they can be dangerous over time. Then I'll outline the Acid Reflux Solution, our easy-to-follow program, which consists of making simple lifestyle changes (many that you can start on today!), altering your diet, and reducing your acid reflux medication, whether you're taking over-the-counter or prescription drugs. As a bonus, if you follow these recommendations and use these recipes on a daily basis, you should begin to notice a gradual but very distinct loss in weight.

To promote your health, in the second half of the book I've included more than 100 delicious, easy-to-fix recipes you can be proud to serve company. These were designed to avoid trigger foods, minimize exposure to common food allergies, and provide portion control. They also include enough fiber to reduce frequency and severity of acid reflux while providing the flavor and culinary satisfaction that will hook you on change. If you use these recipes regularly or follow them as a model in your eating habits, you'll discover a wonderful side benefit: Like me, you will lose weight without even trying, which is absolutely one of the very best ways to alleviate GERD.

By following the healthy eating plan exemplified by our recipes and incorporating the easy lifestyle changes, you will reduce the frequency and severity of acid reflux and feel like a new person. Try it for just a few weeks at first, and you'll see. Not only will bouts of heartburn become less prevalent, but you'll also experience a surge in energy and vitality caused by your improved nutrition. Welcome to a naturally healthy, heartburn-free life!

# PART I

# THE ACID REFLUX SOLUTION

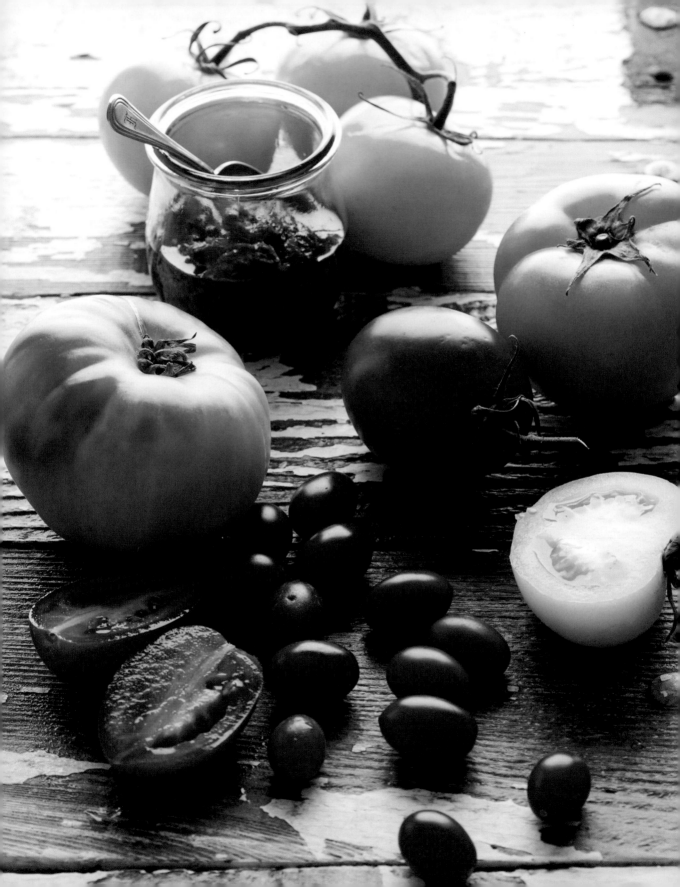

# Chapter I

# ACID REFLUX NATION

*You Are Not Alone*

**IF YOU ARE SUFFERING FROM HEARTBURN,** you are not alone. In fact, you've got way too much company. In the United States, over 50 million Americans complain of acid reflux. That's one-sixth of the entire population. Roughly 44 percent report an attack at least once a week. More than 23 million people experience episodes of heartburn daily. Even for a physician like me, who sees gastrointestinal patients regularly, the numbers appear staggering; but as a person who suffers (or I should say, has suffered) from acid reflux, it is reassuring to know that I am not alone.

What's particularly sad is that this disease distorts one of life's most primary pleasures: eating. Unlike other diseases, you cannot avoid food, one of the primary causes of heartburn. You have to eat—at least three times a day—so it's not something you can ignore. I for one thought paying the price of heartburn after every meal was something I was going to have to do all my life. Happily, I was wrong.

## The Skinny on Acid Reflux

Acute acid reflux, as anyone who suffers from it knows, is a sudden burning surge of stomach acid that flares up into the throat, much like the lava of an erupting volcano. And like lava, it burns everything in its path. The stomach makes acid to help digest food that has recently been eaten. Ideally, that acid should stay in the stomach. But sometimes it shoots up into the esophagus. This is reflux. Reflux usually occurs about an hour after a meal, but it may affect you shortly after you eat. Or maybe it wakes you up suddenly at night hours after you've eaten. I have many patients who swear the accompanying chest pain is so severe they think they're having a heart attack.

We doctors call this sudden, uncontrollable surge of stomach acid gastroesophageal reflux disease, or GERD. Because acid reflux is the primary symptom and major complaint of the disease, the term is often used as a stand-in for GERD. Another frequently used name for the same problem is heartburn, which is most descriptive. For simplicity's sake, we will do the same. In *The Acid Reflux Solution*, you'll find these terms used synonymously along with GERD.

GERD can manifest itself in many ways. Reflux can be so painful that maybe you're afraid to eat. And while obesity is, in fact, associated with GERD, some of my patients avoid food to such an extent that they lose way too much weight, and I worry about malnutrition and their susceptibility to infections. Others lie awake at night, losing valuable sleep time, fearfully waiting for an attack. Worse still, chronic acid reflux causes scarring that produces esophageal strictures, which can make it difficult or even impossible for food to get to the stomach. A further stage of chronic inflammation of the esophagus is a precancerous condition called Barrett's esophagus, diagnosed by a serious change in the epithelial tissues. GERD is even associated with 60 percent of malignant esophageal adenocarcinomas that line the esophagus—the fastest growing cancer in America—that occurs in the area where the esophagus joins up with the stomach.

## Who Gets Acid Reflux?

Though it may seem improbable, GERD strikes people of all ages. Babies, especially those who are not breast-fed, often suffer from acid reflux. You've heard of a "colicky" baby? Well, that colic is regurgitation of undigested milk or formula mixed with stomach acid. The cranky, crying, fussy behavior too often attributed to a defect of personality is an expression of pain.

Young adults are also not immune. At an age when the tendency to overindulge is greatest, we tend to think we're immortal, eating and drinking as if there were no tomorrow. Unfortunately, as anyone who has overindulged at a frat party knows, drinking too much does not come without consequences. How many people have not been woken up by a little bit of acid or bile in their mouth after a long night of celebration? Gross, indeed, but one of the body's early warning signs. If occasional bouts of excess lead to heartburn or even acid reflux, it is usually transitory, and the occasional Alka-Seltzer tablet or swig of Pepto Bismol may be all that's needed. But if drinking—and eating—to excess occurs frequently and continues long enough, heartburn and indigestion can become chronic problems. Symptoms of esophageal discomfort or pain that occur at least once a week can be symptomatic of more serious issues.

People over fifty, though, suffer the greatest frequency of GERD, which may be no surprise. As we age, our bodies lose the ability to compensate, as any middle-aged "weekend warrior" can attest to. The joints don't work as well, and it should be no surprise that our digestive system also undergoes changes with age. Old bad habits, which we can often tolerate in younger years, begin to take their toll. And stress can cause more overeating and too much drinking. Another sad but true fact not to forget is that as we Americans get older, we are prone to getting heavier, and as I mentioned before, overweight and obesity are strongly associated with GERD, something we'll discuss in depth later on.

Two major changes in the population have given rise to the high prevalence of acid reflux. One is the concurrent epidemic of obesity in America. We already know that as a country, we have an issue with food; we love it too much! Let's face it, with 70 percent of the population overweight and one-third of those so obese it threatens not only their quality of life but also their life expectancy, we know something's wrong with the way we eat.

The second major factor contributing to the huge number of people suffering from GERD is the aging of the population. As more and more baby boomers reach the age of sixty-five and the proportion of older adults nearly doubles by 2030 from what it was a decade ago, the proportion of people suffering from acid reflux is going nowhere but up.

## Signs and Symptoms of Acid Reflux

While many older adults suffer from GERD, their symptoms are sometimes less obvious and often more serious. They will attribute a sour taste in the mouth to a touch of indigestion or dismiss chronic dry cough to the air conditioning or allergies. (I know more than one person who went to the emergency room claiming they had a bad stomach flu only to find out their coronary arteries were completely clogged and they'd gotten there just in the nick of time.) Acid reflux can even cause tooth decay and mimic symptoms of ulcers (abdominal pain, nausea) and asthma (coughing, wheezing), causing misdiagnoses and years of unnecessary suffering.

Fully one-third of people who think they have asthma actually suffer from GERD. They develop the characteristic wheezing and difficulty breathing from aspirating acid. Remember that stomach acid we've sometimes tasted after too much partying? At times, the backflow slips down into the lungs, causing irritation that triggers bronchial spasms and other symptoms that are exactly the same as asthma. Once we treat the GERD, the asthma symptoms go away.

Just the other day I had a patient who is a doctor himself. He suffered from severe asthma for three years before his rheumatologist suggested he be tested for GERD. We attached a BRAVO chip (more on this in a minute) to his esophagus and determined that even though he was one of those people who doesn't feel the acid, he was refluxing regularly and severely. In his case, medications did not help, and there was a physical repair needed. Once it was accomplished, his "asthma" disappeared. Amazing, but true.

So how do you know if you are suffering from GERD, or if you're having a heart attack? How can you be sure it's just heartburn?

Possible symptoms of GERD include:

- Frequent heartburn
- Hoarse or raspy voice
- Wheezing and shortness of breath
- Persistent dry cough
- Feeling like you have a lump in your throat or food stuck in your chest
- Difficulty swallowing
- Pitting or discoloration of the teeth
- Feeling full too soon

- Chronic sore throat
- Trouble getting a restful night's sleep

Fewer than half of the more than 50 million people suffering from acid reflux actually seek medical help, usually those who cannot sleep at night. In fact, more than a quarter of all Americans self-medicate for symptoms of acid reflux more than two times a month. But the fact that acid reflux can disguise itself as other diseases is a really strong argument for not diagnosing it yourself. Self-diagnosis usually leads to lack of objectivity. We tend to downplay important symptoms or accentuate minor ones. Diagnosing yourself is a little like trying to fly. If you're estimating the distance below you as only two feet and you're correct, when you take off, you're in the clear. If it's a fifty-foot drop, you're toast.

## Diagnosing GERD

How do you find out for sure if you are suffering from acid reflux? There's a nifty new device called a BRAVO chip. It's a tiny computer and transmitter designed to measure pH, or acid level, which is attached to a microscopic suction cup. The instrument is threaded down the throat of the patient, pressed onto the esophagus, and left in place. The device senses every change in esophageal pH and transmits this information in real time to a receiving monitor secured onto the patient's belt, much like a pacemaker. Basically, it gives the doctor a chart of when and how often the "acid volcano" erupts. It also tells how far the acid travels. A physician like me can read the printout and see exactly if and when acid washes back up into the esophagus. The chip stays there for two days, so that a good picture is relayed of just what is going on during eating, sleeping, exercising, and other activities. After a couple of days, it simply slips off and is washed out to sea, as it were, with the next bowel movement. But by then, I've got all the information I need.

To be sure, not everyone needs a BRAVO chip to diagnose GERD. Quite simply, your physician may decide based on your symptoms alone that you have GERD. But you must be sure it is not a cardiovascular problem that is giving you that pain in your chest in the middle of the night and that you do need the medications you are taking while you are transitioning into your new healthy lifestyle.

Anyone popping even ordinary antacids, let alone powerful proton pump inhibitors, had better be sure they need them. A medical professional should also make sure those antacids are not interfering with other medications or contributing to chronic physiological problems. These pills, while effective, are not benign, and I believe strongly that airing the very real consequences of chronic use may help patients take a closer look at their treatment plan and consider some natural alternatives, such as the ones presented in *The Acid Reflux Solution*.

# Chapter 2

# CLOSE THE MEDICINE CABINET

*More Is Not Always Better*

IF YOU SUFFER FROM ACID REFLUX, chances are you have been taking an antacid medication for some time, whether it's a mild over-the-counter preparation or a strong prescription drug. As a physician, my training involves prescribing medications to treat and cure disease. It's hard to fathom these days, with all our antibiotics and vaccinations, but at the turn of the twentieth century, fully one-third of all deaths in the United States were caused by infectious diseases, primarily pneumonia, diarrhea, tuberculosis, enteritis, and diphtheria. Since the advent of penicillin use in the 1930s, the life expectancy of the average American has risen precipitously. Medications save lives; they cure disease. However, when used inappropriately or abused they not only make health issues worse, but they can also cause disease. Such is the case with most of the medications used to treat GERD.

People with severe acid reflux and ensuing complications need relief, no doubt about that! In severe cases, such as with the precancerous condition called Barrett's esophagus, preventing further damage to the tissues of the esophagus is critical. Even for those with less advanced GERD, repeated bouts of acid reflux can interfere with normal sleep patterns, leading to chronic fatigue and even consequent lowering of immune protection. This can result in greater susceptibility to infections and emotional stress. Some studies even suggest that not enough sleep causes weight gain for a variety of complicated hormonal reasons, leading to obesity. (I don't know about you, but when I don't get enough sleep I am usually ravenous the rest of the next day.) And obese patients suffer from two to three times the amount of reflux as nonobese patients, so weight control is extremely important in GERD control.

The stomach is composed of specialized cells that can withstand the astonishing low pH of the acid that is made there. The esophagus, however, is made of a completely different type of cell, which is more delicate and cannot tolerate such powerful acid without damage. What concerns doctors are the effects of repeated exposure of the lining of the esophagus to that superacidic, corrosive stomach acid with its astonishingly low pH of 1.5. (The lower the number, the stronger the acid.) Considering that your body's natural acid/base balance is a neutral 7.4, that's like taking a blowtorch to the delicate tissues that line your upper GI tract. Ouch!

Repeated exposure to that level of acidity can lead to esophagitis, an extremely painful inflammation that is literally an open sore in the esophagus. Imagine how much any other kind of wound would hurt if you kept irritating it. You know the saying "adding salt to a wound"? In this case, it should be changed to "adding acid to a wound." Ouch, indeed! We can treat esophagitis, but if the irritation continues over time, scarring and development of premalignant or even malignant changes in the cells of the lining of the esophagus can take place. This presents a whole other can of worms.

In extreme cases, pain from severe heartburn and reflux causes some people to avoid food altogether. Dinnertime becomes dreaded, and food the enemy. Some people lose too much weight too quickly; a few actually become anorexic, with serious physiological consequences. Yet human beings are astonishingly resilient; our bodies can compensate for a long time. So if your diet is inadequate, your wonderful immune system and sturdy organs will make up for the abuse they are receiving and work extra hard to keep you healthy. But over time, especially as we age, our bodies lose their capacity to make up for too much damage. Nutrition becomes extremely important as we get older, and not eating a balanced diet because of acid reflux can be extremely harmful. Many of our chronic diseases such as osteoporosis, anemia, diabetes, and cardiovascular disease arise at least in part from poor or inadequate nutrition.

Short-term inflammation, what we doctors call "acute" (though there is nothing "cute" about it), can cause pain and even bleeding. This is where medications really help. However, if the flare-up continues long enough, it is classified as "chronic esophagitis," which is not only painful but also downright dangerous. Many months or years of inflammation and consequent scarring can lead to a closing, or stricturing, of the esophagus. If severe enough, food cannot pass down into the stomach. If enough tissue is affected, it can lead to even more serious consequences. Some medical professionals attribute rapidly rising incidences of esophageal cancer to rising rates of GERD.

So as a responsible physician, I am all in favor of prescribing drugs to quell the symptoms of GERD in the short run. As I said, I've written many prescriptions myself. The problem comes from taking them for too long. Read the package insert: many of these medications are not meant to be taken for more than six weeks in a row; yet people remain on them for years. Extended use can range all the way from over-the-counter antacids that many people pop like candy any time they feel a bit of agita to expensive prescriptions written by professionals like me.

Basically, there are three types of drugs used to reduce heartburn and indigestion:

- Buffers: over-the-counter oral antacids
- Histamine-2, or H2, blockers
- Proton pump inhibitors, or PPIs as they are called

Let's review these so you'll know why they may be helpful until you learn to manage your GERD with the Acid Reflux Solution. But keep in mind that at the end, I'm going to tell you why most people should not take these drugs for longer than a couple of months. (Oh, you've been popping them for years, have you? Well, read on.)

## Buffers: The Acid Slayers

These popular soothers have been around for the longest time. (They neutralize acid that has already been produced.) You know what they look like. Many come in rolls of round lozenges; some in liquid form. Some are pink; some are white. Tums, Rolaids, Alka-Seltzer, Mylanta, Maalox, milk of magnesia, and Pepto Bismol—

which in addition to heartburn, claims to give relief from nausea, indigestion, upset stomach, and diarrhea—are among the most well-known brands.

For a once-in-a-while sour stomach after an unusually spicy meal or too much alcohol, or even with a touch of the flu, these neutralizing buffers—in pill and liquid form—can be just the ticket. Calcium carbonate, which is the active ingredient in many of these remedies, works immediately but lasts for only twenty to thirty minutes. After that, if you've really got GERD, the pain will come bouncing back.

In addition, many older adults consider these harmless and pop them like candy, which some of them resemble. They think they're even good for them because they contain calcium. Some new studies on calcium indicate that too much, just like too little, can be harmful, possibly contributing to heart attacks and fractures. A total of no more than 1,000 to 1,200 milligrams from both supplements and diet is sufficient for most people. Overuse of antacids can be harmful in that they can flood the blood vessels with mineralized calcium. Each Tums Ultra, for example, contains 1,000 milligrams of calcium carbonate. If you pop a couple of these several times a day, you're getting far too much mineral. Best to get your calcium supplement in a prescribed dose and don't overdo the antacids.

## Histamine-2 Blockers

The next most powerful acid inhibitor is a histamine-2, or H2, blocker, also called an H2 receptor antagonist. Specialized cells in your stomach, called parietal cells, secrete gastric acid in response to the chemical histamine-2. The call goes out as soon as the body gets a signal that food is on the way down, especially fat and meat. Smells alone can trigger histamine-2, as well as even the thought or memory of food. Fully 30 percent of stomach acid is secreted via this sort of stimulus. By far the biggest cause of acid secretion, however, is distension of the stomach. The bigger the meal, the more stomach acid is made, which is another reason portion control is so critical for controlling GERD.

H2 blockers essentially intercept or interrupt the signal from the histamine-2 at the beginning, so that the parietal cells remain largely inactive, and much less stomach acid is secreted. These drugs include many familiar names: Tagamet, Pepcid, Zantac, and Axid, as well as less potent over-the-counter versions. They kick in in about an hour and work for twelve hours at the most, but their effectiveness is limited because they do not stop the total production of stomach acid. Therefore, they are most effective for the treatment of mild cases of esophagitis and reflux. It is also important to know that these medications can interfere with other medications, like Coumadin, making it necessary to adjust the dose of those other medications. Another reason for not dosing yourself without telling your doctor.

## Proton Pump Inhibitors

Okay, here comes the big artillery. Proton pump inhibitors, or PPIs as they are popularly called, make H2 blockers look like BB guns. Drugs like Nexium, Prilosec, and Prevacid shut down the acid secretion pathway at the source. They literally prevent the cells from pumping out protons, which are pure acid. PPIs prevent at least 90 percent or more of stomach acid from ever being produced at all. Its action is more delayed, taking up to several hours to kick in, but the effects last for a minimum of twenty-four hours and often up to three days.

If you're suffering from GERD and have constant acid reflux, it's hard to think this might not be ideal. Get rid of the stomach acid, and you eliminate your painful symptoms. That's true. No doubt about it. But it's your long-range health that concerns me, and eliminating acid forever may not present such a perfect scenario. Keep in mind that your body makes stomach acid for a reason. First of all, it properly digests, or breaks down, food so that your small intestine can absorb all the nutrients you need. Initially, protein, starches, sugars, and fats are way too big to squeeze into your body. Acid is essential for metabolizing these large nutrients into smaller molecules so that your body can absorb them and put them to use.

Many minerals, including calcium, iron, and magnesium, cannot be absorbed efficiently without the presence of acid. The acid in the stomach actually changes the electronic configuration of these minerals so that they can be taken up by the gut. You need calcium both for your bones and for your acid/base balance, iron for your red blood cells, and magnesium for the proper function of many muscles, including the heart.

In addition, absorption of essential B vitamins can be inhibited by lack of acid. Vitamin $B_{12}$, in particular, which is a critical nutrient for preventing a very serious form of anemia, can only be taken into the body when bound with something called "intrinsic factor," and shutting down the proton pump often inhibits excretion of intrinsic factor. Also, your body has a certain acid/base balance that is critical to maintain. Your gut contains billions of so-called "good bacteria," which enhance your immune system, aid digestion, and even help produce certain nutrients, like vitamin K.

## Beware of Long-Term Use

Have you ever noticed on that over-the-counter medication you bought that there's a warning not to use the drug for longer than three weeks? I hate to tell you, as a licensed physician, the instructions we receive from the FDA, which regulates all drugs sold in this country, state in very strong language that proton pump inhibitors "should not be prescribed for longer than fifty days." That's a little over a month and a half. How long have you been on your medication? And how many times has your doctor's office handed off a refill prescription without blinking?

Unfortunately in today's busy medical environment, it is sometimes easier to write a prescription for a "benign" medicine than to explore the root cause of the patient's problem. Traditional medicine, in particular, aims very directly at relieving symptoms. But the more we study chronic constitutional problems, like digestive issue in general and GERD in particular, the more we realize that cause and effect may not be as direct as they appear at first glance.

Bottom line: No acid production for a prolonged period of time can lead to poor absorption of many essential minerals and can change the natural balance of your gastrointestinal tract's bacteria. Now can you see why it is not a good idea to use acid-blocking agents for too long a period of time? Too much of a good thing is not always helpful.

According to *The Use of Medicines in the United States: Review of 2010* report by the IMS Institute for Healthcare Informatics, in dollars spent, Nexium was the second leading drug sold in the United States, bested only by Lipitor. Looking at it from another perspective, doctors wrote 53.4 million prescriptions for the generic equivalent of Prilosec in 2010, up from 45.4 million prescriptions in 2009. This placed proton pump inhibitors in sixth place in terms of most popularly prescribed drugs in the United States.

What is the take-home message here? Something that works as well as antacid pills are excellent to quell symptoms while you transition to natural healing, but they should not be used forever. There has got to be a better way for long-term prevention of acid reflux. And there is: the combination of lifestyle and diet we offer in *The Acid Reflux Solution*. Read on.

# Chapter 3

# THE ACID REFLUX SOLUTION

*How to Alleviate GERD Naturally*

**MANY PATIENTS ARE NOT AWARE OF IT,** but there are two schools of medicine at war with each other in the United States. One side, called allopathic, conventional, orthodox, or Western medicine, is the type of health care most of us grew up with, and it's what I was trained to practice. This type of medicine excels at treating symptoms of disease, especially infectious disease, as well as injuries that result from accidents and conditions that require surgery.

The second kind of medicine has a number of names: complementary, alternative, functional, holistic. These differ from each other in that some substitute older traditional forms of healing from other cultures, such Chinese and Ayurvedic medicine, while the complementary medicine I am partial to incorporates natural forms of healing and treatments, such as nutrition and acupuncture, within an orthodox framework. But they all strive to prevent disease from arising in the first place and to get at the root cause of chronic conditions rather than just treating outward symptoms.

It is for good reason that conventional Western medicine became so powerful in the twentieth century, because as discussed in the last chapter, for many years the greatest killers all over the world were infectious diseases like pneumonia, smallpox, typhoid fever, rheumatic fever, polio, influenza, and diphtheria. With the discovery of vaccines, sulfa drugs, and especially antibiotics in the early part of the last century, many illnesses that had wiped out entire populations and decimated families were conquered. This conveyed huge respect and power upon modern medicine and the seemingly simple but powerful pills, potions, and injections it prescribed.

Now that we have gained control over many infectious diseases, we find ourselves faced with new health priorities. Partly because we are living longer and a larger proportion of the population is aging, and partly because of the stresses of our contemporary lifestyle, a new set of diseases is responsible for most of the mortality we face: heart disease, cancer, high blood pressure, stroke, diabetes. Others may not kill us quickly, but cause great suffering and diminish quality of life; these include GERD, or acid reflux, arthritis, obesity, and allergies.

We call these diseases that arise from complex causes and slowly get worse over time "chronic." That is, unlike acute infections, which have a single identifiable cause that usually can be eradicated, these lingering conditions arise from many forces both internal and external working together, and they are not easily treated. Often the treatment of chronic disease requires a mixture of allopathic medicine and lifestyle interventions, such as we offer with *The Acid Reflux Solution*.

As a practicing physician for close to thirty years, I've seen literally tens of thousands of patients and many thousands of cases of GERD. All that experience has tempered my approach to treating heartburn. I believe firmly that for many people, there is a better way to reduce or even eliminate acid reflux besides taking pharmaceutical drugs for the rest of their life. Using proton pump inhibitors for a prolonged period of time is very likely, especially because 30 to 50 percent of patients diagnosed with GERD still report symptoms of acid reflux even with regular treatment on PPIs. You deserve to avoid the potential long-term effects that can occur with chronic use of proton pump inhibitors: anemia, osteoporosis, greater risk of infections, and perhaps even stomach cancer.

## The Program

Believe me, there is a better way that will not only potentially eliminate your GERD and reduce frequency of acid reflux, but will also appreciably improve your overall health. What has worked for my patients—and for me personally—is a combination therapy approach that I call the Acid Reflux Solution.

The program has three parts:

- **Modifying Your Lifestyle:** Easy changes to a variety of physical activities and dietary habits quickly reduce the frequency of heartburn symptoms naturally in just a few days. We list a dozen to begin with. After you've mastered these changes, it's time to begin the heavy lifting.

- **Eating to Avoid Reflux:** Enjoying appropriate portions of the right foods is the foundation of an anti-reflux diet. Very little saturated fat, lots of fiber, and serving sizes that do not stretch the stomach are three of our guiding principles. We also avoid ingredients that irritate and those that trigger reflux in the majority of people. A wonderful side effect of our food choices and serving sizes is weight reduction, which will happen without you even noticing it. Since obesity is the number one preventable cause of GERD, this is a huge benefit.

- **Reducing Your Medication:** Our step-down approach to medication includes reducing dosage and frequency slowly. This is determined on a case-by-case basis and may not be appropriate for everyone. Managing medications requires not only mastering the information in this book but also putting individualized planning in place for your particular situation. A consultation with your physician is essential. Depending upon the primary reason for your GERD, he or she will advise you about how best to reduce antacid medication. People who have GERD with no inflammation or scarring may begin the Acid Reflux Solution immediately. Those with chronic esophagitis, Barrett's esophagus, or a hiatal hernia must work hand in hand with their doctor to make sure symptoms are properly controlled and the disease does not progress. But to avoid the damaging consequences of long-term use of PPIs, a gradual decrease in medication, which must be individualized, should be put in place. If you suffer from Barrett's esophagus or chronic esophagitis, I want you to take this book to your own doctor and tell her or him your plan.

Let's begin with the easy stuff first. I want you to know what you can do to reduce the frequency and severity of your acid reflux almost immediately simply by making small lifestyle changes.

# Twelve Easy Ways to Alleviate Heartburn without Swallowing a Pill

Here are an easy dozen lifestyle adjustments that will reduce symptoms of acid reflux. I recommend you don't do them all at once. Write out a list and think it over. Choose the two or three changes that will be easiest for you to accomplish immediately. Then every week, make a plan to add one or two more healthy improvements to your lifestyle. It's better if you do less and stick with it than overwhelm yourself with trying to do too much.

Whatever you do, do not throw up your hands and quit if you have another attack. Think of how long you've endured the pain of acid reflux. It's going to take more than a few days to return your GI system to its natural health. But you've suffered long enough, so let's examine twelve easy ways to help yourself heal.

## 1. Raise the Head of Your Bed

Let gravity help. You want your upper chest to be higher than your abdomen. Think about it: Most acid reflux occurs during sleep. And it's the kind that bothers people the most. Being woken up by a sudden attack of acid reflux in the middle of the night is extremely distressing, especially when you're in so much pain you think you're having a heart attack. Simply propping up your head with two pillows won't do it. That only bends your neck. Your esophagus must be elevated above your stomach and at an angle that does not put pressure on your throat.

The goal is to elevate the entire head of your bed a minimum of 30 degrees, like a hospital bed. I think the best, and safest, way to do this is to have a firm foam-rubber wedge made, which is inexpensive. Or put a brick under the legs on each side of the head of your bed.

## 2. Eat Less and Eat More Often

Three meals a day are not enough. Doesn't that make you happy? On the other hand, chances are the meals you are eating are way too big. Portion control is absolutely key to resolving GERD. I want you to reduce the size of all your meals, but allow yourself more frequent snacks, and space out your food intake. Go for a modest-size breakfast, lunch, and dinner, with two small snacks in between whenever you get hungry. What's most important is cutting down on the amount of food in your stomach at any one time. Sixty percent of gastric acid production is caused by stretching of the stomach. If you start using our Acid Reflux Solution recipes (beginning on page 62), you'll begin to get a good idea of portion control, because they have been tailored for this purpose.

Remember in the last chapter we learned that one of the triggers for release of acid is distension of the stomach. To avoid this, practice eating only until you are barely satiated. Do not let yourself get full. Some of us are so used to shoveling in all kinds of food mindlessly—not just meals, but chips, fast food, fries, and candy, not to speak of stretching out our gut with literally gallons of soft drinks—we can't even remember the sensation of being just perfectly satisfied.

If you think this may be one of your issues, pay attention when you eat. Some professionals use a kind of chart labeled from one to ten. The very lowest number, one, indicates that you are famished. You haven't eaten in three to five hours, your blood sugar is low, and you're crashing. The highest number, ten, signifies you are absolutely stuffed and could not eat another bite if you tried. Now, the idea is two-fold: You don't want to wait until you're starving to eat; that's just going to make you eat more than you need to. And for some people, extreme hunger can trigger an attack.

By the same token, you don't want to stuff yourself, which will both add weight and increase acid. The key is to improve your sensitivity to hunger and satiety. Get to know your body better and what it really needs. And remember always, less food means less acid reflux. Eat only until you feel you have had just barely enough. Always leave room for a little bit more.

This is easier when you know that a tasty snack is waiting for you. You don't have to stop eating; you just have to eat less at any one time. When planning meals, if you'd like soup or a salad first, be sure to reduce the size of your main course portion even further. And, of course, I've got some ideas about *what* you should eat, but we'll get to that later.

## 3. Drink Before or After Meals

To minimize pressure on the stomach and the lower esophageal sphincter, or LES, the circular muscle charged with keeping all the acid and partially digested food in your stomach, reduce volume by drinking as little as possible with your meals. Take your beverages, preferably water or herbal tea, at least half an hour before you eat. Or wait thirty to forty-five minutes after you eat to drink. That way, your stomach won't get distended enough to call for more acid. It's not just the volume of what you drink; think about how the liquid affects dry foods, causing them to expand. The combination of popcorn and apple juice, for example, could blow up to three times the initial volume. Ouch! It hurts me just to think about it. Best to separate solids and liquids, just like recycling bottles and cans.

Now, from being a practicing physician, I know that beverages are a loaded issue. Many Americans are used to downing literally gallons of soft drinks a day. I'm sorry to be the one to tell you, but if you want to get rid of your GERD, that's just going to have to stop. For one thing, all that liquid distends your stomach, resulting in your feeling the need for more food to fill you up at mealtime and increasing the release of stomach acid. Second, carbonated beverages are a trigger for acid reflux, whether it's soda or beer. And last, whether sugar-sweetened or sugar-free, all these carbonated drinks are associated with greater obesity—the leading cause of GERD.

## 4. Chew Your Food Well

If you tend to wolf down your meals, make yourself count to a minimum of twenty with each bite. Keep in mind digestion begins in the mouth. When you chew and get a chance to really taste the food, your salivary glands secrete saliva to moisten it and form what we call a bolus, the wad of moist food you swallow. At the same time, enzymes are released that start the digestion of complex carbohydrates and some fats. If you don't chew your food well, you skip this stage of digestion, which just makes it harder to deal with further along. The whole process of digestion involves breaking large molecules down into smaller and smaller molecules until they are tiny enough to enter the body via the gut.

## 5. Loosen Your Belt

There are several other ways to remove pressure on the stomach. One is to wear loose-fitting clothes. It's no joke. A belt that's too tight or a waistband that cinches in your abdomen reduces the room you have for food, increasing the pressure on your stomach, which can trigger the release of extra acid. It also stresses the lower esophageal sphincter. Make it as easy as possible for everything to pass right through. No problema. What's a smart-looking pair of sweats for, anyway?

## 6. Sit Up Straight

You have to consider your physical position. When eating at the table, watch your posture and sit up straight. Okay, you've been hearing that since you were a kid, but now it's really important. Slouching and folding your abdomen in half is the same as wearing a belt that's too tight. If you're a TV watcher, make sure you don't hunch over a coffee table to eat your dinner. Otherwise, I promise you, it's going to come back at you sooner rather than later.

Sitting up at the table also forces you to confront your food. Look at it, appreciate it, savor it, and know that there are no seconds. What is on your plate is what you are going to enjoy, so take the time to appreciate it.

## 7. Eat Slowly!

Give your digestive system a chance to work. It takes roughly twenty minutes for your body to send signals of satiety, a measure of fullness, to your brain. If you take smaller bites and have a conversation—with your significant other or your dog or cat, it doesn't matter—while you're eating, you will eat less in a longer time and probably enjoy it more. When you're just shoveling in the calories while watching TV and paying no attention to your plate, you are likely to eat far more than you should. If you allow time for the body to signal it's comfortable and has had enough and if you pay attention to your own cues, you will naturally eat less and feel more satisfied.

## 8. Remember Gravity

It's just common sense not to bend over after eating. An inverted posture invites reflux. If you drop something, leave it there; it will wait. Do your exercises beforehand. I'll even take it a step further and recommend you don't lie down, even if you are tempted to, for at least thirty minutes after a meal. Forget about that postprandial siesta. If eating makes you a little tired, resist the temptation to take a nap right after lunch or dinner. Instead, take a little walk, even just around the block. You will be astounded at the good that will do for your digestion.

For one thing, like shaking a sieve, the act of walking upright helps jiggle everything along, so that your meal passes through your gut physically. On top of that, the movement of your leg muscles—and your arms if you swing them—stimulates the absorption of glucose from your food into your cells. This can help a lot, especially if you are insulin resistant or have type-2 diabetes. It's one reason exercising helps people lose weight.

## 9. Don't Eat within Three Hours of Bedtime

For me this is the golden rule. Even if I've been doing really well for days—or weeks or months—if I forget myself or get carried away at a party and chow down after nine o'clock, invariably I'll spend a miserable night suffering from acid reflux. This can be challenging for people who like to stay up late, because at a certain point you're going to crave a midnight snack. What can I say? We all have choices to make, and this may be yours. If you get really hungry and absolutely have to eat, have a few soda crackers, just enough to take the edge off.

## 10. Move It or Lose It

According to the latest government recommendations from the Centers for Disease Control, adults age twenty-one to eighty-one all benefit from $2\frac{1}{2}$ hours of moderately vigorous exercise or $1\frac{1}{4}$ hours of vigorous exercise a week teamed with a weight-bearing exercise session twice a week. In fact, the older you are, the more you benefit. If there is any real secret to eternal youth, it's remaining active.

Now the good news is that this requirement of thirty minutes of exercise five days a week can be accomplished in ten-minute intervals, as long as you get your heart rate up. For example, if you park your car at the far end of the parking lot at work or at the mall and walk briskly to your destination, preferably taking the stairs, you might easily get in one ten-minute session. You'll get a second when you return to your car. So now all you have to do is be creative for the third session. And the weight-bearing exercise does not have to be weight lifting. Gardening and yoga can qualify, as long as you are stressing your muscles.

Okay, here's the bad news. Really vigorous exercise beyond a certain point with the accompanying hyperventilation (aka panting), can actually put enough pressure on the LES so that it releases and allows a surge of acid. Marathon running, for example, is out. On the other hand, low physical activity paired with obesity has been associated with greater prevalence of hospitalization for symptoms of GERD. So I recommend strongly that you do establish some regular pattern of physical activity, but especially starting out, restrict your cardiovascular exertion to a moderate amount. If you work with a trainer, let him or her know your issues. Walk before you run.

The truth is, though, unless you are a saint or superhuman, if you're not exercising now, it's very difficult to start, let alone to pack in thirty minutes a day. And you are unlikely to overdo it. I know because I've been there. And the truth is, the heavier you are, the harder it is to move: bulk makes motion more awkward.

So here's my advice. Take it from someone who dropped 30 pounds in the past year. Do whatever you can as long as it is more than you were doing before. Build up gradually and be kind and forgiving of yourself. Pick an activity that you enjoy, you can afford, and is easy and convenient enough that you will stick with it.

For me, it turned out to be exercising and weight lifting at a gym. And it doesn't have to be a fancy gym. Many YMCAs have fabulous exercise programs and well-equipped weight rooms. For my colleague Susan Wyler, it was yoga. For you, it could be a walk with a friend. Walking the dog is not a good choice, because unless you have it well trained, it's going to stop to sniff the grass every two feet, which will not do you any good. Cycling, swimming, tennis, dancing, gardening, even house cleaning are options. Anything that will make you stress your muscles and move your limbs as well as get your heart going provides beneficial physical activity.

What does all this talk of exercise have to do with eliminating GERD? Bottom line: It's going to help you lose abdominal weight, and that lessening of pressure will relieve your heartburn.

## 11. Reduce Stress

Even we doctors debate about how much stress contributes to digestive problems. For years, ulcers were blamed on psychological and emotional stress—until it was discovered that many ulcers are caused by bacterial infection. It's really hard to know whether stress and acid reflux coexist with each other or whether one is responsible for the other. What I can say is that if you are stressed, you are going to be more sensitive to any symptoms you do have, and probably bothered by them to a greater degree.

In terms of acid reflux, reducing stress is, of course, most important if you are one of those people who overeats when they are nervous, or if you are someone who doesn't eat at all when you are stressed. Because either way, it's going to make your symptoms worse. Stuffing yourself and starving yourself can both trigger bouts of painful reflux.

Relieving stress is easier said than done, I know, especially if the problem involves work or your social life. But you can learn to manage it. I think you'll find that taking a stand and doing something for yourself is a good first step. Look around and see what resources are available that you feel comfortable with: counseling, yoga, meditation, a ballroom dancing class, amateur theater. Anything that takes you out of yourself can help. Even talking with a friend. Sure, these recommendations are cursory and simple, but they are a good start. Find something that you enjoy and are passionate about and pursue it! It's good for your heart, and your heartburn.

## 12. Quit Smoking and Cut Back on Alcohol

Now I'm beginning to sound like a preacher, but as a physician, I have to say it. Both smoking and excessive alcohol consumption cause GERD; it's as simple as that. So it's up to you. If you're taking the Acid Reflux Solution seriously and you really want to get rid of your heartburn, you've got to stop smoking. Nicotine is a major reflux trigger—period.

Alcohol is a little more forgiving. Excessive drinking will definitely trigger reflux. But personally, I don't see a problem with having a glass of wine with dinner if you are not in an inflammatory state, especially if you get a little food in your stomach first.

So there you have it: a dozen great ways to alleviate or even eliminate acid reflux with small physical changes and healthier lifestyle choices. But there's one more factor that cannot be ignored: diet.

# The Acid Reflux Solution No-Diet Formula

Both *what* you eat and *how much* you eat contribute greatly to GERD. What you eat determines whether your problem is triggered or not; the amount influences your weight status. Eating too much at one time can trigger acid reflux. In addition, it inhibits weight loss. And as I've said before and I'll say again, carrying around too many extra pounds is probably the single most predictive indicator for frequency and severity of acid reflux. So rather than constantly quelling symptoms by taking too much medication for too long and chipping away at your body's reserves, it makes sense to remove the problem that is causing those symptoms—particularly acid reflux—in the first place. And the way to do that is to eat right.

Because eating a healthy diet is a big part of the Acid Reflux Solution—and difficult for so many of us to actually start and maintain—I've dedicated the rest of the book to describing exactly why and how to eat in a way that can reduce acid reflux. The benefits of the lifestyle modifications suggested above will accrue as you integrate them into your daily routine. When you start eating a healthier diet on top of the lifestyle modifications, you should start to see a pretty dramatic reduction in your acid reflux symptoms. Hopefully, you will consult with your doctor at this point to reduce the dosage and/or frequency of the acid reflux medication you take over time.

For people who need to slim down in the first place, losing even just 5 percent of your weight—that's 8 pounds if you weigh 160, for example—will greatly improve your health in general. And most will find, as I have, that losing 10 to 15 percent of body weight completely eliminates GERD. For people who are normal weight or even underweight and still suffer acid reflux after following the Acid Reflux Solution and adopting our anti-reflux recipes, there is probably a genetic or chronic physiological reason for it, and some ongoing medication or possible surgical intervention may be necessary. If you have intractable GERD, you may want to consult the appendix, Medical Technology to the Rescue, page 195. There you'll find more clinical options that can help.

## Reduce Your Medications

Not long ago, I made a business trip to Miami, which gave me the opportunity to visit my mother. She planned an elaborate Cuban dinner, and I approached with a big smile of anticipation on my face. As soon as she opened the door, however, I was shocked. My mother looked unnaturally pale and sick. After much cajoling, I finally convinced her to see her physician. A few days later, she called me with the diagnosis: she was extremely anemic with a hemoglobin (red blood cell) count that was half of normal. Other blood tests revealed that she was very iron deficient. Thankfully, her work-up did not uncover any hidden malignancy or source of internal bleeding. What the doctor's visit did reveal was that my mother had been taking proton pump inhibitors daily for years, which had prevented her from absorbing the iron she needed to make new red blood cells. (She is going to be the first one to get a copy of this book!)

So my own mother is the perfect example of how eliminating or greatly reducing stomach acid can adversely affect your ability to absorb essential minerals like iron and calcium. But what do you do if you suffer from heartburn or acid reflux and have been using antacid buffers, H2-blockers, or proton pump inhibitors daily more than the recommended six weeks to prevent unwelcome symptoms from occurring? If you have been placed on treatment with any kind of antacid— whether H2-blockers or proton pump inhibitors—by a physician, and you have been taking the prescription for more than six weeks, you should definitely follow up with your provider to see why you are still on medication. Let your physician know you want to get off the pills and tell him or her about your intentions to make some serious lifestyle changes. Regardless of the response, if you want to heal yourself naturally, you can still follow the Acid Reflux Solution. For most people, it is simply not appropriate to be on treatment for GERD indefinitely.

First, try out as many of the easy lifestyle modifications (see page 24) as you can; these will immediately begin to alleviate some symptoms. Then make the commitment to change your eating habits. If you follow our recipes and the portions suggested, you will automatically begin to lose weight. If you really want to ditch those medications, try to avoid snacking, sugar-sweetened beverages, and desserts whenever possible. After you've lost 5 to 10 percent of your body weight or you have been symptom free for three weeks, try stopping the medication and see what happens. If you have some acid reflux but it's not as acute or it's less frequent, you may want to resume your medication or taper off while you continue the lifestyle adjustments and diet for another month or so and try weaning yourself off them again. If your symptoms still persist at that time, consult your health-care provider.

If a doctor was never involved, you didn't receive a formal diagnosis, and you took it upon yourself to start over-the-counter antacids, you can stop taking them at any point. There is no accepted way to stop these medications. They are not addictive, so you do not have to taper off. However, if you have not modified your diet and weight, you will probably notice symptoms of GERD as soon as you stop taking them. So, my suggestion is to follow our plan and lose weight as I just described for two months, then stop your antacids but keep them on hand. Take them as a palliative measure only when you are actually experiencing heartburn, not because you anticipate an attack. If your symptoms persist even after you have lost 5 to 10 percent of your usual weight, then definitely consult with a physician because something other than GERD may be occurring.

So now that we've gone over the dozen simple lifestyle changes that will alleviate acid reflux and explained why changing your diet and reducing your medications is so important, let's look at what the Acid Reflux Solution says you can eat and what you should avoid. What's on the menu may surprise you.

Chapter 4

# WHAT'S ON THE MENU?

*More Than You Think*

SINCE I'VE PROMISED YOU an anti-reflux eating plan, you are probably eager to learn just what is on the menu. Keep in mind, the Acid Reflux Solution is not a formal diet but a lifestyle plan that includes information on healthy eating to alleviate GERD paired with more than 100 recipes that contain ingredients and cooking techniques helpful for preventing acid reflux. In this chapter you'll learn which foods are most likely to precipitate attacks, but more important, the wide variety of foods you can enjoy even if you have been diagnosed with GERD. You'll also find out why fat is such a problem, why portion control is critical, and why natural, unprocessed foods are the best choice. You will also learn the importance of understanding why fiber is an exceptionally important part of an anti-reflux diet. Finally, we'll touch on a couple of ingredients that are natural aids to digestion.

Now, we get to the meat of the matter (no pun intended): what you can eat that will not bring on an attack of painful acid reflux and what you cannot. The reason I think you're dreading this discussion is that if you've purchased this book, you've probably read at least two or three others, which suggested a very limited diet. While the choices the Acid Reflux Solution allows in general may pleasantly surprise you, deciding exactly what you can and cannot eat may not be as simple as you'd expect. That's because of the individual differences we all experience. Wouldn't it be nice if someone could just hand you a list of foods to avoid so that you'd never have an attack of acid reflux again? Believe me, as a doctor who wishes all good things for his patients that would be my fervent wish. I'd say simply, "Don't eat X, Y, and Z," and you'd never endure a painful bout of heartburn again. Unfortunately, it's a little more complicated than that.

But let's start with the common lore. Most materials on heartburn and acid reflux say essentially the same things: You can't eat tomatoes—there goes your favorite Italian food. You can't eat highly seasoned or spicy food—there goes Mexican, Indian, and Thai. You can't eat citrus fruit, vinegar, or raw vegetables—oh, no, there goes salad! What's left to live for?

What if I told you there is no scientific evidence any of these prohibitions are necessary or that following those rules will eliminate symptoms of GERD? Remember, we learned that acid reflux is caused when the LES, or lower esophageal sphincter, the circular muscle that acts as a gate between your esophagus and your stomach, loosens too easily or does not maintain its tone, so that the caustic gastric acid escapes into your esophagus. Very few foods can actually pry open that valve.

## Foods to Avoid

Researchers have done studies with many foods, literally measuring the reaction of the LES with a tiny electronic instrument lowered into the esophagus, where it monitors how the muscle responds when individual substances are swallowed. Many such studies have been conducted with a grocery list of foods, and while it may seem surprising, only a few substances actually cause the LES to relax. The list includes:

- Mint and anything containing mint oil
- Chocolate
- Saturated fat
- Processed meats, like bacon and bologna
- Deep-fried foods
- Carbonated beverages
- Caffeine
- Coffee, whether caffeinated or not

- Alcohol
- Nicotine (granted this is not a food, but it is a major chemical trigger)

As you can see, there are fewer than a dozen substances scientifically proven to trigger GERD. If you suffer from acid reflux, you definitely should not eat or drink (or smoke) anything on this short list. Scientific studies have proven that some of these foods, like chocolate, mint, and caffeine, chemically cause the LES to loosen, triggering acid reflux.

Other foods that are greasy or high in saturated fat lie heavy on the stomach and slow digestion, delaying the passage of food through the GI tract, which

## Eat Like an Italian

When it comes to Italian food, some books say just don't go near it. So how do you account for the fact that most Italians eat pasta every day; some eat it twice a day—and they're not avoiding tomato sauce. Yet their incidence of reported heartburn is only 14.8 percent compared with 38 percent in much of northern Europe and 42 percent in the United States. How can that be? Well, one reason is that they eat small portions. Pasta is almost always enjoyed as a separate course in Italy, very rarely as a main course. If you check out our recipes, you'll see that a portion of pasta consists of only 2 ounces. I guarantee you'll be able to enjoy that with no difficulty. But have seconds or pile on the 4 ounces (uncooked) that most of us consider a fair portion, and you'll be up all night.

Second, traditionally in Italy just enough sauce is added to coat the pasta lightly. Spaghetti is never served swimming in sauce the way it is here. Nor

is it stuck together with gobs of cheese or washed down with gallons of soda and half a dozen greasy garlic knots. Most important, dinner often begins with a small antipasto, usually of vegetables—think salad—and cooked vegetables are served with the meal. Dessert, if offered at all, is usually fresh fruit. Think fiber. Finally, after they eat their meal, the family gets up from the table, goes outside, and takes an evening stroll. Think about how moderate physical activity aids your digestion.

I love pasta and pizza and as I've told you, I suffered from acid reflux. So if like me, you can't imagine giving up these wonderful foods for life, here's my solution—eat like an Italian:

- Small portions
- A modest amount of sauce or gravy
- A light sprinkling of cheese
- Lots of vegetables = high fiber
- Take a short walk after eating

causes a kind of traffic jam. Things back up higher on the line, which precipitates a buildup of pressure on the LES, which can loosen it and initiate acid reflux. Meats high in saturated fat, especially processed meats, fatty cheeses, and fried foods are at the top of this list. So I urge you to eat red meat less often and in much smaller portions. Forget about those 8- to 12-ounce hunks of beef served up at tony restaurants. Those days are gone—good-bye. Remember the doggy bag—even if that dog is you the next day. At home upon occasion, a 3- or 4-ounce portion of lean red meat, such as loin of lamb or beef fillet, served with a salad and vegetables may do you good . . . or not. You'll find out how much you can take. And definitely, take your dinner at lunchtime, or have supper early so your body has time to digest the meal before you lie down.

You must cut way down on processed meats like bacon, sausage, bologna, salami, corned beef, and pastrami. If you're serious about getting rid of your GERD, you really should take these foods off the table. You don't have to give up milk and cheese and yogurt, but choose lower fat versions where possible and/or enjoy smaller amounts. You'll find the sharper the cheese, the less you need to eat to enjoy the flavor. That's why I often suggest pecorino Romano over Parmigiano-Reggiano or just a sprinkling of pungent feta.

Deep-fried foods are extremely hard to digest and most likely to initiate reflux. Particularly for my readers who live in the South, where everything is fried and barbecue is king, I know this is a hardship. But believe me, it's worth the effort to transform your preferences. It will just take a little time. Think about switching to leaner ways of cooking that call for less fat, butter, or oil. Grilling, broiling, baking, and poaching are fine alternatives. Marinating meat and chicken or dusting them with a dry rub are good ways to pick up extra flavor with less fat.

As a last thought, beware of processed foods. They are filled with chemicals designed to delay degradation and extend shelf life, and they may have hidden ingredients that do not agree with your GERD. Now, compared to what you've read elsewhere, that isn't really such a long list, is it?

## What You Can Eat

Why aren't tomatoes prohibited, you ask? What about citrus fruits? There's an important distinction here. These are acidic foods, not trigger foods. You might also wonder about spices, which most other books say to avoid. These could be classified as stimulant foods. Let me explain. If you are in the middle of an acute inflammatory stage and you have esophagitis, a painfully irritated esophagus, it's just common sense you'll want to choose bland foods and avoid acids and spices. Not because they would cause reflux, but because they will acerbate your discomfort. This is the time you may need to consult your doctor and turn to medications to quell your symptoms for a few weeks until you feel better.

But most of the time, if you are not in pain or suffering from obvious symptoms of frequent reflux, except for specific trigger foods like chocolate and coffee and general foods like saturated fats and processed meats, your shopping list is wide open. Variety is an important part of a healthy diet. At the same time, the key to natural healing with the Acid Reflux Solution is to choose foods that will improve your digestion and reduce both the frequency and the strength of heartburn attacks. This means lean meats, chicken, and fish; as many natural unprocessed foods as possible; and plenty of fiber from an assortment of fresh fruits and vegetables and whole grains.

## Portion Control Is Key

The truth is, most of the time it's not so much what you eat as how much that determines whether you'll suffer from heartburn that night. Think about it. One excellent article I read noted that people often complain about the spicy food they eat giving them GERD, when it is really the quantity of the food they eat that sets off their reflux. When are you more likely to stuff yourself: at the Indian buffet or when you're eating a tuna salad sandwich at your desk? When that Mexican combination plate is set in front of you, with enough food to feed three cowboys, or when you're keeping your grandmother company and picking at salt-free chicken and potatoes.

## Natural Foods Are the Best Foods

How you cook as well as what you prepare also affects digestion. Instead of frying, try roasting, grilling, or poaching. As a rule, substitute extra virgin olive oil for butter or margarine. Look for reduced-fat sour cream, cream cheese, and yogurt. Or opt for goat's milk dairy products, which contain less fat and many find easier to digest than cow's milk dairy. I don't like nonfat dairy products. If you read the label, you'll see they sound more like chemistry experiments than food.

Buy organic whenever you can. While studies of the nutritional benefits of organic over conventional produce are controversial, they do show that you ingest less pesticide residues with organic. Likewise, so-called organic, free-range chicken and meats are leaner, and the fats they do contain are of a completely different complexion than those of feedlot animals. They have less saturated fat, and what they do contain is higher in anti-inflammatory omega-3s in relation to inflammatory omega-6s, producing a healthier ratio of these fatty acids. If you can afford it, go the extra mile and pamper your gut as much as you can.

In a similar vein, using organic flours, grains, and soy means you avoid GMOs, or genetically modified organisms. Much of our country's wheat and corn crop contains genes you would not expect to find in a plant. Now, I'm not saying that's what's causing our epidemic of GERD. As I've said, I think the number one reason is the epidemic of obesity. But I am suspicious of what insecticides and fish genes inside plant genes do to our immune systems.

In Europe, there are very few genetically altered foods on the market, because the European Union has decided that the chemical manufacturers and growers must prove these crops are safe before they are sold for human consumption. Here in the United States, on the other hand, corporations are allowed to introduce genetically modified foods first—planting them in fields and delivering them to the consumer fresh or processed—and they are removed from the marketplace only if and when the USDA, FDA, or EPA can prove they are dangerous. Since it can take decades for cancer to develop and it is often difficult to pinpoint the etiology of autoimmune and chronic systemic diseases, it's going to take a long time before we know whether these altered foods are totally benign. My feeling is that it only makes sense to play it safe and opt for fresh, organic fruits, vegetables, and meats wherever possible.

## How to Encourage Natural Healing

It's easy. The mantras I'd like you to adopt are:

> *Portion size, portion size, portion size*
> *Fiber, fiber, fiber*

These two elements are probably the most important aspects of an anti-reflux diet. Portion control will go a long way toward liberalizing your diet. You may not tolerate eating an orange, but you certainly can—and should—risk a teaspoon or two of lemon juice in your vinaigrette. You might even tolerate half a fresh orange. The vitamin C will do you a world of good, though believe me, you can get plenty of ascorbic acid from other vegetables that star in our recipes, like cabbage and sweet red peppers. One serving of a tasty dish like our Spanish Chicken and Rice (page 130) will feel great. Seconds will do you in. Less quantity overall relieves pressure on your stomach, reducing secretion of stomach acid.

At the same time, a higher proportion of fiber will keep what you do eat moving right along. However, you don't want to overdo it, or you'll produce gas, which can be uncomfortable. Start using the Acid Reflux Solution recipes, many of which include generous amounts of fiber, and you'll get an idea of what a proper anti-GERD portion looks like.

## Why Fiber Is Your Friend

Fiber is the part of fruits, vegetables, and whole grains that is hard—or impossible—to fully digest. Ironically, this same quality improves our digestion. Some fibers draw moisture into the gastrointestinal tract; others add bulk and move everything along. Certain fibers act as feed for the good microbes in our gut that actually nourish us and improve our health.

Fiber is an extremely important part of the Acid Reflux Solution. Why? To put it bluntly, chronic constipation is often associated with GERD, and fiber helps promote regularity. It keeps everything moving along regularly as it should. Let's be real, there is no genteel way to discuss bathroom habits. But discuss them we must. Think of your GI tract as a train track. The lead train loads up, filling with passengers, and chugs out of the station, carrying them along to their destination. Each train departs at a certain interval. Maybe the schedule says one train every twenty minutes. Usually there are a number of trains on the same track, but in different places at any one time. As long as the lead train keeps moving, all runs smoothly and efficiently. But if one of the trains breaks down and can't get to the final terminal, all the trains behind it back up on the track, causing congestion. Other cars get stuck in the tunnel, and passengers about to board start crowding around on the platform, spilling over onto the stairwells. If you think of it that way, it's not surprising that GERD is often associated with chronic constipation. Plainly speaking, fiber keeps the trains running on time.

Partially digested food moves out of your stomach and journeys as briskly as is appropriate down the twenty-five to thirty feet of your intestinal tract. But when that system clogs, pressure and gasses build up closer to the stomach. Like the physical pressure of abdominal fat, this distension causes the LES to relax, making it more likely to allow a bout of reflux. Many reasons exist for constipation, but when we examine patients who complain of being irregular, certain common habits are prevalent. We find theses patients often do not:

- Drink enough water
- Walk enough
- Ingest enough fiber

Now I know I told you not to drink too much fluid with your meals. That's because portion control and volume are critical. You don't want to build up too much pressure in your stomach during meals. But that doesn't mean you shouldn't drink plenty of fluids in between. In fact, as we age, our need for water becomes greater while at the same time our thirst tends to diminish. This means we can begin to become dehydrated without feeling thirsty. If you're an active person who exercises a lot, you'll probably sweat enough to build up a thirst. Where have you seen an athlete without a water bottle? Whether thirsty or not, the average adult requires a minimum of 1½ to 2 quarts of fluid a day to remain properly hydrated. The key is to keep on sipping water slowly throughout the whole day.

Notice, I use the word water. Not diet cola, sugar-sweetened soda, beer, coffee, or juice. Remember, carbonated beverages, including beer, are major triggers of acid reflux. And for most people, so is coffee, whether caffeinated or not. Colas are high in phosphates, which create an acidic environment in your system. Aside from leaching calcium from your bones and contributing to osteoporosis, this acid may trigger heartburn beyond what you'll get from the volume of the carbonation alone. Many juices, especially orange juice, are also highly acidic. Plain pure water and herbal tea are the best choices to quench your thirst and satisfy your body's need for fluids.

My recommendation is to fill your water bottle or thermos in the morning and refill it in the middle of the day, if needed. If you don't already own a water bottle, go to the store and pick one out you really love—one that's a pretty color or smart looking or just plain cool. These days everyone drinks water in public. Take frequent small sips but slow down after meals, even if you feel a little thirsty. Drinking too much right after eating can put excessive pressure on the stomach and trigger an attack. If you enjoy a cup of hot tea after dinner, wait half an hour or so after eating to make room for it.

Keep in mind that digestion actually begins in your mouth, continues in your stomach, and delivers its biggest benefits in the intestines, mostly near the top. That's why it's so important to chew well before swallowing. Your body has been alerted dinner is coming down the pike, which causes the gallbladder and pancreas to release digestive juices mixed with powerful hydrochloric acid made in the stomach. Your body secretes 1 to $1^1/_2$ quarts of these juices everyday. Within a few minutes of hitting the stomach, whose powerful acid registers a pH of 1.5 on a scale of 10 (remember, the lower the number, the stronger the acid), all that food turns to mush, or as we professionals call it, chyme.

So now you've got a wet mass of highly acidic sludge sloshing around in your tummy. It wants to pass on to your small intestine, where the acid will be neutralized by other secretions rich in bicarbonate, otherwise known as baking soda—the same stuff you swill to get rid of the pain when you have heartburn. Soon a great deal of water from this sludge is reabsorbed into the body as most of the nutrients are absorbed. The kidneys also filter out water and either reabsorb it back into the body if it is needed or excrete it as urine. But if you are dehydrated or chronically low in fluid intake, that mass passing through your lower GI tract can dry out too much and get stuck. The train has left the station but has encountered a problem!

What do you do when you have something caught in a tube, like trying to get ketchup out of the neck of a jar? You shake it, of course. Gravity is your first line of attack against congestion—or constipation. Remaining upright and moving after a meal not only helps prevent stomach acid from spurting up into the esophagus, but it also keeps everything moving down. And when you walk, the motion helps shake the contents further along. Movement actually stimulates peristalsis, the involuntary waves of contractions you don't feel, which is how the intestines pass their contents down the line. The custom of taking a leisurely stroll after dinner, which is particularly popular in Italy, has an excellent basis in healthy digestion, and I highly recommend it. It's a great way to get at least some of the thirty to forty-five minutes of exercise we all need every day.

In addition to taking advantage of gravity, shaking everything down the system, walking also stimulates the movement of energy into your cells. This is especially helpful if you are overweight or obese and suffer from insulin resistance. Exercising your muscles as you walk opens up a back door for the energy to reach your cells, even if the front door is stuck. When your cells get what they need from the food you eat, the body has less of a tendency to hold on to excess or even to produce more energy of its own.

So drinking too little and remaining immobile both contribute to constipation. Drinking enough and walking even a little bit every day help keep you regular. The third major factor in avoiding constipation is fiber. Think of fiber as nature's sponge. It draws water from your body into the colon and by doing so keeps things moving and less likely to become constipated.

Fiber is key to regularity. Here's my short course on how to get what you need: eat lots of fresh fruits and vegetables and sufficient though not excessive amounts of whole grains. Also make sure you have moderate amounts of nuts. What do I mean by "lots" and "sufficient"? Have at least one whole fruit at breakfast; juice doesn't count. This could be a banana, an orange (or even half an orange), a chopped-up apple, diced mango, an apricot, or a peach. Or maybe $1/2$ cup of berries on your oatmeal or cold cereal. Or a modest wedge of papaya or melon, with or without a small scoop of low-fat cottage cheese. You can also enjoy a piece of fruit as a snack between meals. Just remember not to eat any raw fruit within three hours of bedtime.

For vegetables, go for at least four different nonstarchy vegetables a day, both raw and cooked. If you're talking about leafy green vegetables—such as lettuce,

## Regularity First Aid

Sometimes with the best of intentions, what we prescribe doesn't work. If the good advice I gave you above does not do the trick, there are other ways. Prune juice is high in sorbitol, a natural so-called "sugar alcohol" in the body that does not affect glucose levels and so is not used for energy. Instead, it draws moisture into the intestines and can function as a very effective laxative. Just don't overdo it: $1/2$ cup should be enough, twice a day, if necessary. Studies have shown that prune juice is more effective than many over-the-counter laxatives at alleviating constipation. Another trick is to sprinkle 1 tablespoon of wheat germ over your oatmeal or cold cereal or stir it into $1/2$ cup of applesauce. One or the other of these two—or both if you're really in need—are most likely to do the trick.

arugula, spinach, kale, broccoli, chard, collards, cabbage—you can eat as much as you like, but choose an assortment and not more than 1½ cups total at any one time. To prevent reflux, remember to restrict volume, always. Remember: too much of even a good thing is still too much.

Many other vegetables are essentially "free": cauliflower, zucchini, green beans, orange winter squash like acorn and butternut, sweet potatoes, eggplant, fennel, asparagus, artichokes . . . enjoy them all. They are free because they should not contribute to GERD, and they contain very few calories. Avocadoes do have more oil, but it is a very healthy fat and full of vitamins, so I heartily endorse them in moderation. (How could a Cuban not?)

Starchy vegetables such as white potatoes, corn (really a grain), and peas should be eaten with more discretion and not as frequently. Beans are a really good source of fiber, but as everyone knows, they can cause gas, which we want to avoid at all costs, so only a little—½ to ⅔ cup max—at a time.

A few vegetables are especially difficult to digest and should be avoided. These include jicama and Jerusalem artichokes (sunchokes) as well as raw onions and garlic, except in very small amounts. They contain a complex chemical called inulin, which is an insoluble fiber that is normally beneficial but which produces a lot of gas in many people. I recommend staying away from them completely. However, modest amounts of cooked onion or garlic should not trigger GERD in most individuals, and garlic offers some benefits to your immune system.

Many books have a much longer list of vegetables to avoid. We've already discussed tomatoes. I'll be very surprised if many people actually have a problem with an appropriate amount of fresh ripe tomato. Or even a modest amount of tomato sauce, especially the lighter sauces you'll find in this book. Tops on many lists of taboo foods for people suffering from acid reflux are the vegetables that tend to "repeat": namely, onions, garlic, bell peppers, especially the green ones, radishes, and cucumbers. Do I agree? Yes and no.

For best digestion and to avoid constipation, you need a mix of soluble and insoluble fibers, which you get from beans, vegetables, fruit, grains, and nuts. Soluble fiber absorbs moisture and softens the stools so they are easy to move. Insoluble fiber stimulates the smooth muscle of the intestinal walls so everything moves along nicely. This fiber also provides a nice meal for the good bacteria living in your large intestine, which modulate your immune system, help produce vitamin K, and metabolize certain essential fatty acids.

In addition, fruits and vegetables provide great natural sources not only of fiber but also of vitamins, minerals, and antioxidants. Remember, whole food is almost always better than a supplement. Unless you really overeat, which some do with fruit, it's hard to take in too much fiber. But many people with digestive issues can have problems with insoluble fiber. In general, oats are easier to manage, so I usually recommend them first to my patients. A small bowl (½ to ⅔ cup) of oatmeal in the morning with ½ cup of fruit and low-fat or soy milk is a great way to start out. Quinoa, a whole grain that is very rich in protein, is also easy to digest.

Wheat is a little trickier. In addition to fiber, doctors and nutritionists recommend whole grain and especially whole wheat products because they are naturally rich in iron, potassium, zinc, and many essential B vitamins and often fortified by manufacturers. But while the nutrition content of whole wheat is much higher than refined, large amounts of whole wheat or wheat berries, or even spelt, can be hard for some to digest and can trigger acid reflux. That's why I recommend white rather than whole wheat pizza dough. The same may be true of brown rice.

Some people even have trouble with too much pasta, which is refined wheat. In fact, a lot of times, people think it's the tomato sauce that's getting to them, when it's really the pasta. If you're one of them, try eating a modest portion, no more than 2 ounces before cooking, which is the portion given in all our pasta recipes. I think you'll be pleasantly surprised.

In fact, my advice for all grains is to experiment a little and see what your body tolerates comfortably. Your first line of defense is to cut the amount you eat. This applies particularly to whole wheat and brown rice. If that doesn't work, then you may have to avoid a particular grain. If you don't eat enough whole grains, make sure you take a supplement or get your nutrition from enriched cereals.

So it may seem counterintuitive to think about one end when you're worried about the other, but take my word for it, avoiding constipation will help alleviate GERD. Here's my prescription:

- Drink more. At least 1½ and preferably 2 quarts of water or herbal tea a day. Sip it slowly throughout the morning, afternoon, and early evening.

- Move more. Take a short walk every evening after dinner. Half an hour is ideal, but twenty minutes will offer great benefits. Or take a ten- to fifteen-minute stroll after lunch and another short walk after dinner.

■ Eat more fiber. The average adult man needs about 38 grams of fiber a day; the average woman, 25 grams.

## Special Foods That Aid Digestion

In addition to all the foods we've already discussed, there are a few ingredients that are considered aids to digestion. Ginger and fennel are two of these, and you'll see them figure prominently in our recipes. Sailors have long known the calming digestive effects of ginger, which we use fresh, dried or glacéed (candied), and even pickled. The Chinese have touted its digestive benefits for centuries. A recent article published in the *European Journal of Gastroenterology and Hepatology* documented why ginger is so helpful for digestion. The researchers found that it speeds up the passage of food from the stomach into the beginning of the small intestine. We call this "increased motility," and it's what you want to encourage, especially when you suffer from GERD.

Fresh fennel is a delightfully crisp high-fiber vegetable that can be eaten raw or cooked. Anecdotally, it is said to relieve bloating. Fennel-Scented Lentil Soup (page 91), Rosemary-Fennel Chicken Cutlets (page 134), and Baked Flounder over Fennel Niçoise (page 113) are just a few of the mild anise-flavored dishes designed to soothe your stomach. Dried fennel seed, a sweet spice, packs even more punch.

Now that you know what generally constitutes a GERD-friendly diet—what triggers acid reflux, what seems to prevent it as well as what other factors are helpful—I think it's time to explore how all these rules and regulations pertain specifically to you. Let's explore our differences.

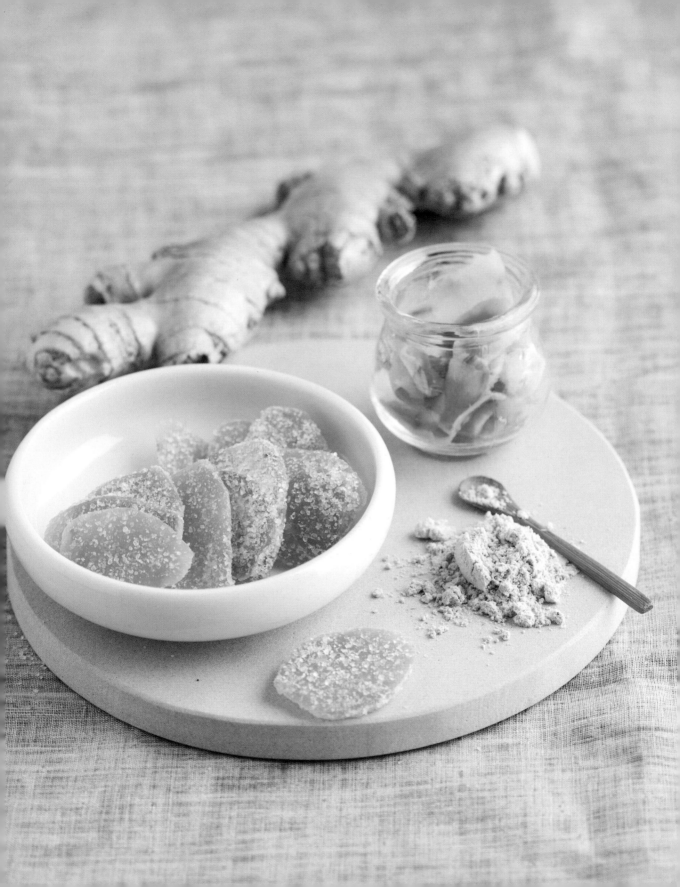

# Chapter 5

# EVERYONE IS SPECIAL

*Making the Acid Reflux Solution Work for You*

**OKAY, NOW THAT I'VE TOLD YOU** everything you can eat, including many delicious foods you thought were taboo, I want you to tell me what you can't eat, or at least what you may not want to eat. The truth is that after an exhaustive search of the medical literature, there is still professional disagreement about whether certain foods cause GERD or not. Particular ingredients affect some people and not others; diet is very individual. So now that we've given you our do's and don'ts list that works for the majority of sufferers, I want you to make a personal record of which of these foods—or any other foods—affect your acid reflux the most. Because no matter what I tell you about the science of GERD or what has or has not been proven, you're more sensitive and knowledgeable about your digestion than anyone else. No matter what I say, you know which particular foods set off your acid reflux.

I can tell you that if you peel your sweet peppers and cucumbers and remove the seeds, they should be much more digestible, and that there is no scientific evidence they trigger reflux. Yet you might throw them in a salad and curse me that evening. I can explain all the statistics about the Italian diet and tell you how with appropriate portions, you should be able to enjoy a plate of pasta with tomato sauce. But you might take me at my word and end up feeling as if Mt. Vesuvius were erupting right inside your stomach.

With all the patients I've seen over the years, the differences in tolerance of various foods astounds me. One person cannot stand tomatoes at all, even though the acid in tomatoes does not cause the lower esophageal sphincter, which seals off the stomach, to relax. Another person can eat fresh tomatoes, but not canned, which makes a little more sense, since extra acid is often added to canned tomatoes for food safety.

How can it be that I tell you something is perfectly fine to eat, with no evidence it is related to GERD, yet for you it triggers reflux? That's because every human being is unique, and various nutrients in foods affect individuals in very unique ways. The "rule" we used to develop the recipes in this book, and the parameters for what was included and what was excluded, were based on the latest scientific studies. But these results often pertain to statistical majorities—what works for most people. There is nothing that is guaranteed to work for all people.

## It's in the Genes

We all have a set of genes that contains our DNA and determines who we are and to some degree how we are. Think of these genes as a book, and the DNA as a formula written on the pages, which tells every cell in the body what to do and when to do it. Only thing is, unlike our alphabet, this genetic code is written in only four letters: G, C, A, T. But when that DNA is passed down to us, sometimes the transcriber makes a mistake. She puts a G where there should be a C, for example, or vice versa. One little error can lead to very big consequences.

Every single one of us has about fifty thousand of these tiny "misspellings," called Single Nucleotide Polymorphisms (SNPs, pronounced "snips"). Sometimes we never find out about these little blips. Many of them don't affect us at all. Some are in parts of the DNA that are inactive or have no visible effect. But a few may occur in regions that control how we metabolize nutrients, and that is what makes us unique. Maybe everyone else in the room needs the equivalent of only one orange to get all the vitamin C they need for a day. But for a person with a particular SNP, the equivalent of three oranges might be needed. Since they wouldn't want to eat three oranges, this person might need a vitamin C supplement. Another SNP may not allow someone to absorb vitamin $B_{12}$, leading to a condition called pernicious anemia. These people may require vitamin $B_{12}$ injections for the rest of their lives.

## Food Allergies Play a Role

Likewise, some people can eat all the bread and pasta and crackers they want; others cannot tolerate wheat at all. Celiac disease is a genetically programmed intolerance to gluten, a protein that occurs in significant amounts in wheat, barley, and rye. People with this genetic variation recognize this protein as something foreign and try to get rid of it. Unfortunately, the body mistakes a similar protein in the small intestine for the gluten protein and tries to get rid of that protein by inflaming the small intestine. What a horrible case of mistaken identity! This severely impairs the lining of the small intestine, which is a very important place for nutrient absorption. Damage to this part of the intestines leads to problems with fat digestion and vitamin and mineral malabsorption, and it can also slow passage of food through the gut. Consequently, many people with this malady report serious acid reflux.

Other symptoms of celiac disease are not as obvious: iron-deficiency anemia that has no known cause, which can lead to extreme fatigue, and poor calcium absorption, which can lead to premature osteoporosis, to name just a few. The damage done to the lining of the gut often results in lactose intolerance, as well. What is really interesting, though, is that symptoms resolve completely on a gluten-free diet.

Because many people have either celiac disease or a similar gluten intolerance that does not have the genetic marker, and they don't even know it, and because so many people with the problem suffer from GERD, it's worth trying a gluten-free diet for a couple of weeks to see if it alleviates your symptoms. The only trick is that you have to be very strict about it—no cheating. And you have to play detective, because there is gluten hidden in many products you would not suspect.

Begin by eliminating all wheat, barley, and rye. Oats are usually tolerated in small amounts, but try giving them up as well just to see what happens. Also taboo are beer and many processed foods that contain either wheat or hidden sources of gluten. If you want to try a gluten-free diet, you're going to have to become an expert at reading food labels. Beware of ingredients called modified food starch, modified vegetable starch, natural flavors, caramel coloring, hydrolyzed vegetable starch, dextrin, malt, and maltodextrin; they are all code words for ingredients that contain gluten. Even antacids often contain fillers and binders that contain gluten.

While the number of people with actual celiac disease is relatively small, the number of people who have become intolerant to wheat has grown significantly in recent years, nearly one in a hundred at present. What causes this is not clear. Is it a SNP that affects a large portion of the population? Is it a gene they are inserting in our genetically modified crops or residue from a particular insecticide? Why have so many people suddenly lost the ability to tolerate an important source of protein?

## Don't Overlook Hidden Food Allergies

These kinds of food allergies are not the kind that call for a skin test. Those allergies stimulate the release of histamine; they are acute and highly inflammatory, causing rashes, swelling, sneezing, sometimes even difficulty breathing. Instead, think of these as intolerances, because they act on the part of the immune system that lies inside the gut, and their action is more subtle. Any damage occurs more slowly over time, usually taking three to four days to manifest, and you may not connect the food with the reaction—which could range from a headache to acid reflux.

The most common foods that trigger these kinds of food allergies, or intolerances, are wheat, cow's milk (along with cow's milk yogurt, ice cream, and cheese), eggs, and nuts, especially peanuts. They are intolerances developed during the first eighteen months of our life, when the lining of the gut is very permeable. Except for intolerance to wheat, none of these other intolerances has been shown to cause acid reflux. But if you suspect you may have a problem, it's easy to test. Simply stop eating that one food for two to three weeks, and see whether there is any change in your digestion. If there is, remove that one food from your diet. But make sure you consult your doctor or preferably a registered dietitian, who is a licensed nutritionist, to make sure you are getting all the nutrients you need. If you avoid a major food completely, you may need a supplement.

In addition to your particular ability to digest specific foods and any possible hidden food allergy, there's one other very important factor that will determine which recipes work for you and which don't. And that is how you feel at the moment. Has your disease been quiescent for some weeks? Or are you in pain? Is your esophagus inflamed or not?

## A Does Not Always Equal B

If you've suffered from GERD for any length of time, chances are there have been periods, for reasons not always obvious, that the disease has flared up. When the reflux of caustic stomach acid into the esophagus occurs often enough, it causes redness and inflammation, just like any other major irritant. Since you cannot see whether your esophagus is inflamed, you must rely on your symptoms to suggest whether you have active esophagitis, which is not usually subtle. Most likely, you'll feel a persistent burning under the lower end of the breastbone, also known as the "xiphoid process." Food or liquids may burn as they go down the esophagus. Some patients can even trace the path of their food. When GERD is active, it's just common sense to avoid anything that could act as an irritant: spices, vinegars, and acidic foods. Plus, this active period is the perfect time to use antacid medication . . . for a limited time.

On the other hand, sometimes we avoid foods that we think triggered our heartburn, but they were just innocent bystanders. What do I mean by that? One summer evening, when I was seven years old, we had a cookout, and I had a big slice of watermelon for dessert. It turned out that I had the flu and shortly after eating the melon I threw up. Let me tell you, it took years before I could enjoy a wedge of watermelon again. You may well associate tomatoes or spicy food with an attack of acid reflux that was triggered by something different entirely, but the two occurred at the same time, so you logically put them together as cause and effect.

When deciding which foods to include and which to avoid, keep an open mind and take into account how you feel at the moment. Just because you could not tolerate vinaigrette dressing on your salad two weeks ago does not mean you cannot now. When deciding what parameters to use for our recipes, we raised the bar pretty high on digestibility and reflux relief. Paramount are portion control to relieve pressure and fiber to keep everything moving right along.

So make your own personal list and when you check out our scrumptious recipes at the end of the book, skip any that you think will give you problems, at least for the time being. Because I'm willing to bet that if weight is a factor in your health, what is true of your digestion today may well not be true in six months after you've followed the Acid Reflux Solution.

Because while this was designed primarily as an eating plan to alleviate acid reflux, not to lose weight, the two are related. If you follow the plan, reduce saturated fat, and maintain portion control, you will lose weight without even trying.

So please do me a favor. Unless your reflux is very bad, every time you lose five pounds, try one of the foods you think is a trigger for you, and see when it finally disappears. I have confidence that over time, you will be able to enjoy many foods you thought were out of bounds forever. Now, if that is not a solution for acid reflux, what is?

Chapter 6

# WEIGHTY MATTERS

*How to Eat Well (and Lose Weight) on This Program*

**BEFORE WE GET TO THE RECIPES**, let's review *The Acid Reflux Solution* so far. We've gone over the "mechanics" of acid reflux and talked about how prevalent it is, with almost one-sixth of the population of the United States reporting some symptoms. If you suffer from GERD, you are not alone. Almost 50 million Americans share your pain. We've discussed all three categories of medicines—simple antacids, histamine-2 blockers, and the powerful proton pump inhibitors—explaining how they offer excellent options for quelling symptoms and healing when your esophagus is raw and inflamed. However, we've cautioned they do not provide a cure and can have serious health consequences if used for years.

In place of chronic dependence on antacids, particularly the PPIs, I gave you my Acid Reflux Solution, a sensible combination of diet and lifestyle accommodations, which can permanently alleviate the symptoms of GERD. Twelve lifestyle interventions were offered, one of which is moderate exercise. Next, we detailed just what you can eat and what you can't. One of the biggest changes in diet is a reduction in fat, especially saturated fat. This means omitting or greatly reducing ingestion of fried foods, red meats, processed meats, and other processed foods that are high in fat. We also explained how to eat, including posture, dress, time of day, proper chewing, number of meals, and most important, portion control. To prevent acid reflux, it is essential to avoid stretching out the stomach and to limit intake.

So, we concluded, if you follow these recommendations, even if you don't experience a total cure, your reflux will most likely occur less often and be less severe. Now let me point out one bonus of the plan that increases the likelihood of success. Our recipe for success includes:

- Regular moderate exercise
- Much less fat
- Portion control

Can you guess the bonus benefit?

## Effortless Weight Loss

If you follow the Acid Reflux Solution, gradual weight loss will be a wonderful side effect, and you don't need to plan it. No counting, no diet restrictions. It will just happen, and you won't have to work at it. For most people, it takes eliminating roughly 500 calories a day to lose a pound a week. When you think of it, this is a very easy number to achieve, especially since my plan does two things: it significantly reduces both fat and the size of portions.

Of all the foods we eat, fats are packed with the most calories—more than twice that of protein foods, starches, and sweets—so cutting back on fats is the easiest way to remove calories from the diet. Foods that contain a lot of sugar and no other nutrients are other easy ways to reduce. Since carbonated beverages are a reflux trigger, substituting water or herbal tea for sugar-sweetened beverages will easily save you 200 to 300 calories a day.

Eliminating processed meats like sausages and salami, which are laden with fat, as well as processed convenience foods, like breakfasts on a stick and pop-up pastries, each of which contain roughly 200 calories, will buy you the rest you need. So will switching from red meats and fatty cuts to lean meats like chicken and turkey and eating more fish. As for portion control, it is vital. Eating even just one-third less than you ordinarily do can easily deduct anywhere from 150 to 300 calories.

If you skip breakfast, you'll just eat more later in the day. The truth is, people tend to fill out their usual number of calories one way or another. But if each time you eat you have to be careful of the amount, over time you will be satisfied with less, you will become more attuned to your body's "satiety cues," when it tells you you've eaten enough, and you'll be happily satisfied with the delicious recipes we offer. The high fiber content of many of our recipes, which contain plenty of fruits, vegetables, and whole grains, will also make you feel fuller than empty sugar calories that spike your blood sugar and offer no protein and little in the way of micronutrient support—that is, vitamins, minerals, or antioxidants. You'll slim down without working at weight loss, and as your weight issues resolve, so will your reflux.

## Why Weight Matters

The fact is, obesity is a major cause of acid reflux. In fact, it's the single most preventable risk factor for GERD. As I've told you, I experienced the connection myself. Until a couple of years ago, I was technically obese my entire adult life, and I suffered from GERD, though until recently, I didn't put the two together. The truth is, I didn't think about my weight a lot. I'm a fairly tall man, and I carried it well, as they say.

What's more, with more than two-thirds of the American population overweight, and almost half of those people obese, it's hard to keep perspective on what a healthy weight looks like. Even many of our favorite celebrities are overweight, if not obese. All along, I just thought I was normal. I looked like everybody else. Consequently, no matter how painful that nightly acid reflux, I didn't think too seriously about losing weight because I didn't believe I had a problem (or at least that big a problem), and I didn't connect the two conditions. This from a doctor who should know better.

## What Is a Hiatal Hernia?

A hiatal hernia occurs when the top of the stomach pushes up past the diaphragm, bulging over the top. It's not uncommon and is often associated with acid reflux. Medications as well as many of the lifestyle recommendations you'll read about in

*The Acid Reflux Solution* will help. But if the hernia becomes enlarged and symptoms too severe, a laproscopic operation called a Nissen fundoplication (see page 200) can repair the damage and cure the acid reflux permanently.

I calculate body mass index (BMI) in my patients all the time. BMI is a relationship of height and weight that has been proven over time to correlate with life expectancy and health risks for chronic diseases, like diabetes, high blood pressure, cardiovascular disease, even some forms of cancer. You can go online, Google "BMI," and an automatic calculator will come up; just plug in your height and weight. A normal healthy person has a BMI that can range anywhere from 18.5 to 24.9. Overweight is 25 to 29.9. Obese is a BMI of 30 or greater.

When I started working on this book, my BMI was 31.4 —not just overweight, but technically obese! As a doctor, I already knew extra weight was a risk factor for GERD (not to speak of all those other diseases I just mentioned). You see, if there's too much excess abdominal fat, the stomach is pushed in and up, but it has nowhere to go. Like a corset, it literally squeezes the stomach, forcing it where it doesn't belong, leaving the contents nowhere to go but up. That pressure sometimes results in a hiatal hernia, where the stomach slips up past the diaphragm and into the chest cavity. Only the esophagus belongs in the chest cavity, not the stomach.

Other times the big squeeze just exacerbates existing reflux. When it's that tight, something's got to give. With me, starting to write this book and my frequent television appearances on shows like *Today*, *The Doctors*, and *The View* made me more conscious of my weight. When I began incorporating the Acid Reflux Solution recipes as a regular part of my diet and taking my own lifestyle advice, I found the pounds started disappearing while all I was thinking about was getting rid of my acid reflux. Talk about fringe benefits!

This inspired me to take it all to the next level. It did occur to me that appearing leaner would be better for my television appearances. And if I gave the talk, I had to walk the walk. I started going to the gym—regularly—doing a mix of cardiovascular exercises like the elliptical trainer, which got my heart rate up and stimulated my metabolism, and weight training, which is fabulous for building muscle and maintaining healthy bones.

Even then, it did not occur to me that this would make such a big difference in my life. But it did. One day I woke up, and my GERD was gone. Even though it shouldn't have, it took me by surprise. After all those years, to be able to eat with relish, and lie down relaxed, unafraid of those late-night attacks was like a dream. I realized that not only was healthy weight loss a side effect of our recipes, but the mere act of losing weight was also the best medicine there was to fight acid reflux.

Keep in mind you don't have to be "the biggest loser" here; whatever you do will help. Even dropping 5 percent of your body weight can have dramatic positive effects on your health. Not only GERD but also diabetes, high blood pressure, and often cholesterol respond to this kind of moderate weight loss. Five percent of 150, for example, is only 7½ pounds. Five percent of 200 pounds is 10 pounds. If you can lose 10 percent, all the better. But keep the focus on how you feel and on enjoying what you eat every day. Food needs to become your friend, but not the friend that you cling to for salvation, running to for comfort whenever something is wrong. That's an unhealthy relationship. Food has to be the type of friend that sustains you and makes you better. As with any good relationship, you want it to be there for life. So don't think of these helpful hints as temporary solutions. They are a way of living from here on.

Now I'm aware that some people reading this book may have suffered from severe GERD for so long that they are afraid to eat. That's the flip side of this awful disease. For certain individuals, the pain is so severe and the fear of that sudden reflux so great, they actually become anorexic. Being too skinny can also have very serious consequences for your health, especially for women, who are susceptible to iron-deficiency anemia and osteoporosis—both exacerbated by long-term use of antacids, especially proton pump inhibitors, like Nexium, Prilosec, or Prevacid. Acid in the stomach is very important for the correct absorption of iron and calcium. So if for years you have stopped the production of stomach acid, it should be no surprise that for years your absorption of iron and calcium has been compromised.

By following the healthy eating plan exemplified by our recipes and incorporating the easy lifestyle changes, you will reduce acid reflux and feel like a new person. Not only will bouts of acid reflux become fewer and farther between, but you'll also experience a surge in energy and vitality caused by your improved nutrition. Try it for just two weeks at first, and you'll see.

## How to Eat

While *The Acid Reflux Solution* offers a way of eating, not a formal diet plan, there are some tips I'd like to offer about how to structure your meals.

### Breakfast

We didn't include breakfast recipes here because the morning meal is a very personal choice. That's fine. Just three caveats: don't skip it, reduce the sugar and fat content, and as usual, watch your portion control. Many people are under the misconception that breakfast is a great time to reduce calories just by skipping a meal. Or they say they don't feel like eating when they wake up. Believe me, studies have shown that people who eat breakfast are leaner than those who don't. If you don't eat in the morning, your body will nudge you to make up the usual number of calories you eat later in the day, which means a bigger meal in the afternoon or evening. This means a greater chance your body will not be able to use those calories for energy all at once and more food than usual will be converted to fat. At the same time, the greater volume increases the chances of acid reflux.

Another reason to eat in the morning is to jump-start your metabolism. When you skip a meal, your body assumes you are sick or cannot obtain food. It goes into retention mode and slows down your metabolism to make sure you won't starve if the deprivation lasts. So even if you don't feel like it, get in the habit of eating something healthy in the morning—a small container of light yogurt and perhaps a single slice of whole-grain toast. Choose a piece of your favorite fruit over a glass of juice. If you like cereal, that's a good healthy choice. Choose one that is low in calories, which usually indicates less sugar and fat, and make sure you put your portion control into action. Use a measuring cup to dish out whatever the box says is a single portion, usually ⅔ or ¾ cup—not a whole cup. Add 1 percent or 2 percent milk, soy milk, or rice or almond milk. Or opt for one egg, poached or cooked in just a small amount of butter in a nonstick pan, or a single pop-up waffle or small portion of pancakes. Skip the bacon and sausages or allow yourself one small piece.

## Lunch and Supper

For lunch, consider half a sandwich and a tossed salad, or one of our tempting main-course salads like Buffalo Chicken Salad with Blue Cheese and Light Ranch Dressing (page 104) or Greek Salad with Chickpeas and Feta Cheese (page 100). Or opt for a comforting soup like Scallop-Corn Chowder (page 88) or Carrot Bisque with Ginger Cream (page 81). We've got quite an assortment to choose from. If you practice portion control, you can enjoy pasta. Yes, even Spaghetti and Meatballs (page 151) or Orrechiette with Broccoli Rabe, Ricotta, and Sausage (page 146).

If you are willing and able, consider taking your major meal at noon. Eating heavier earlier in the day is much better for your digestion, because you are up and about, letting your food go down all the way before you retire for the night.

When planning meals, leaf through our chapters on soups, salads, poultry and meats, seafood, vegetables, and pasta, rice, and grains. You'll see the amazing and delicious variety of foods you can enjoy while doing yourself a big favor. Many of the main courses are also designed to deliver extra fiber along with protein. For example, Herb-Crusted Rack of Lamb (page 140) is served atop a scrumptious ragout of white beans. Pistachio-Crusted Salmon (page 119) is baked on a bed of tender green cabbage. Even Savory Mini–Meat Loaves (page 144) are studded with oats and corn.

For meaty recipes that stand on their own, such as Asian Barbecued Chicken (page 128), Shrimp-Stuffed Tilapia (page 123), and Salmon Filet Mignon with Herb Butter (page 122), plan your menus so that you include at least one leafy green or other nonstarchy vegetable and a grain on the side. When composing your plate, aim for one-quarter meat, fish, or chicken; more than half the plate green or orange vegetables; and the rest a starch: grain, pasta, rice, or potato.

And for being so good to yourself, a couple of times a week, choose one of our tempting desserts designed to treat you without tripping you up: White Chocolate Mousse with Raspberry Swirl (page 188), Cocoa Meringues (page 191), Pecan Tea Cookies (page 192), Apple Coffee Cake (page 181), and more.

So now that you know how to begin the Acid Reflux Solution—with easy lifestyle changes and a reduction in your medication—you're ready to advance to the pleasures of healthier eating. The recipes that follow are all designed to make it easy for you to reduce heartburn, lose weight without trying, and enjoy every bite.

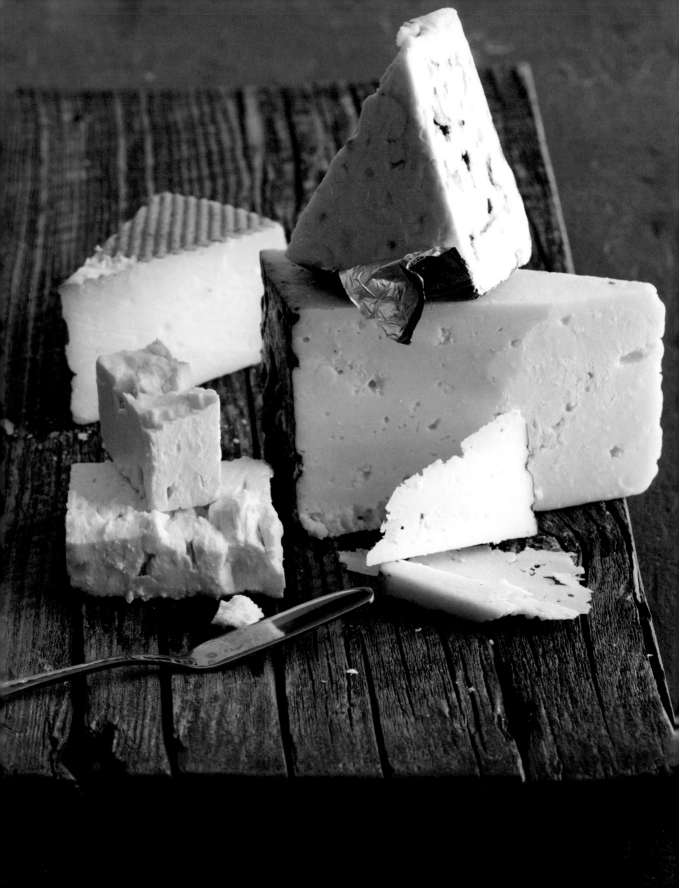

# PART II

# THE RECIPES

# APPETIZERS AND SNACKS

# Babaganoush with Pomegranate Molasses

Makes about 2$^1$/$_2$ cups; serves 6

Many babaganoush recipes are too acidic and garlicky for us GERD suffers. This one enhances the flavor with tart-sweet pomegranate molasses, which you can find in the Middle Eastern section of many supermarkets or in a Mediterranean market, and it incorporates just a whiff of garlic. Enjoy your babaganoush with carrot or zucchini sticks, lightly steamed cauliflower, or sweet red pepper strips.

2 medium eggplants ($^3$/$_4$ to 1 pound each)

3 tablespoons tahini

1$^1$/$_2$ tablespoons pomegranate molasses

1 tablespoon freshly squeezed lemon juice

1 clove garlic, crushed

$^1$/$_2$ teaspoon ground cumin

$^1$/$_4$ teaspoon Aleppo pepper

1$^1$/$_2$ tablespoons extra virgin olive oil

2 tablespoons chopped fresh cilantro or parsley

Sea salt to taste

Prick the eggplants in several places. Either roast over a hot fire in a barbecue grill (my favorite way) or in a 425°F oven, turning several times, for 35 to 45 minutes, until the skin is blackened and the eggplants are very soft. Cut in half, scoop the insides into a bowl, and mash with a fork, or scoop the eggplant into a food processor.

Add the tahini, pomegranate molasses, lemon juice, garlic, cumin, Aleppo pepper, and olive oil. Blend well; if using a food processor, pulse until fairly smooth. Stir in 1$^1$/$_2$ tablespoons of the cilantro and season with salt to taste.

Transfer to a serving bowl and sprinkle the remaining $^1$/$_2$ tablespoon cilantro on top.

NOTE: Aleppo pepper is a wonderful mildly hot pepper with good flavor, which makes a nice stand-in for the spicer varieties. If you think you cannot tolerate any heat at all, substitute freshly ground black peppercorns.

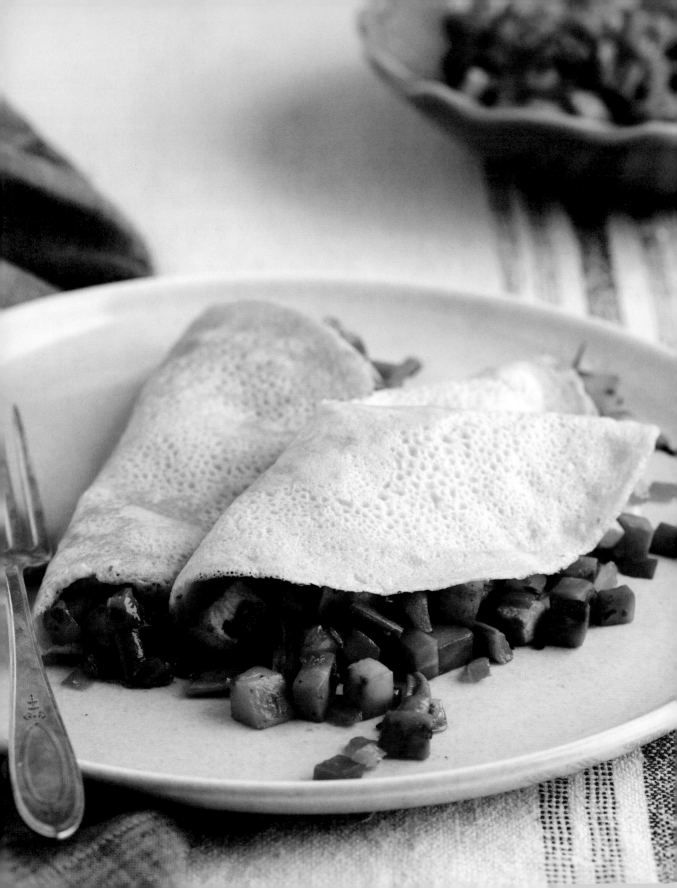

# Mediterranean Chickpea Crepes

Serves 4 as a light main course, or 6 as a starter

In the south of France, they make these crepes, called *socca*, as large as a pizza, with only chickpea flour as a base. I blend it with bread flour and just one egg and make smaller, easy to manage crepes in a skillet. These are unbelievably light, delicious, and digestible. Any kind of cooked chicken will work here: roasted, poached, or grilled. I often pick mine off a leftover rotisserie chicken. I prefer French green beans, called haricots verts, for this dish because they are small and tender.

12 Chickpea Crepes (recipe follows)

1 yellow onion, chopped

2 tablespoons extra virgin olive oil

$1/2$ cup finely diced Yukon gold potato

$1/2$ cup finely diced carrot

$1/2$ cup sliced green beans, preferably haricots verts

$1/2$ cup finely diced zucchini

1 cup diced cooked chicken

$1/2$ teaspoon herbes de Provence

Salt and freshly ground black pepper

Make the crepes and set aside.

In a 10-inch skillet, cook the onion in the olive oil over medium-high heat, stirring occasionally, for 3 to 5 minutes, until golden. Add the potato, carrot, green beans, and zucchini. Cover and cook, stirring once or twice, for 3 to 5 minutes longer, until the vegetables are tender.

Add the chicken and herbs, toss to mix, and warm through. Season with salt and pepper to taste.

To serve, scoop about $1/3$ cup of the filling onto a crepe and either roll up or fold over. It's fine if some filling spills out.

## CHICKPEA CREPES

Makes about 12

1 cup chickpea flour

$1/2$ cup organic bread flour

$1 1/2$ tablespoons extra virgin olive oil

$3/4$ teaspoon salt

2 cups cold water

1 egg

Combine all the ingredients in a food processor or blender. Blend until well mixed.

Heat a 7-inch nonstick skillet or lightly oiled crepe pan over medium-high heat. Ladle in about 3 tablespoons of the batter and cook for $1 1/2$ to 2 minutes, until golden brown on the bottom. Flip over and cook for $1 1/2$ to 2 minutes longer, until the second side is spotted brown and the batter is cooked through. If the crepes start cooking too fast, reduce the heat to medium.

NOTE: These can be set on a plate at room temperature with squares of waxed paper in between to prevent sticking for up to 3 hours; reheat in a low oven if you like.

# Black Bean and Corn Salsa with Cilantro and Lime

Makes about 2¹/₄ cups; serves 4 to 6

Colorful and bright-flavored, this chunky salsa makes a great dip for corn or vegetable chips. It also livens up simple grilled fish and chicken. And it can be added to a composed salad on a bed of crisp greens.

1¹/₂ cups canned black beans, preferably organic, rinsed and drained

³/₄ cup cooked fresh or canned corn

¹/₃ cup diced piquillo or peeled roasted red bell pepper (see note)

2 tablespoons chopped fresh cilantro

1¹/₂ tablespoons chopped scallion

2 teaspoons freshly squeezed lime juice or rice vinegar

1 tablespoon sunflower or peanut oil

¹/₄ teaspoon ground cumin

Salt and freshly ground black pepper

In a medium bowl, combine the black beans, corn, bell pepper, cilantro, and scallion. Toss the salsa gently to mix.

In a small bowl, whisk together the lime juice, oil, and cumin. Season with salt and pepper to taste. Drizzle over the salsa and toss to coat lightly.

NOTE: Piquillo peppers come in jars and offer a nice piquant but not hot note. Otherwise, ordinary peeled, roasted red bell peppers, which are available both jarred and in olive bars in many supermarkets, would do nicely.

# Chickpea Poppers

Makes about 3 cups; serves 8 to 10

Throw out those fatty chips and cheesy doodles that put you at risk for an attack. You won't miss them at all when you whip up a batch of these tasty and nutritious nibbles. Put out a bowlful for a cocktail party or sprinkle on a handful to enliven any simple salad. If you make them ahead, they'll keep well in the refrigerator for up to 5 days, though they're best at room temperature or warm. While these can become addictive, remember portion size—no more than 1/3 cup at any one time.

1/2 pound dried organic chickpeas (about 1 1/2 cups)

1 tablespoon extra virgin olive oil

1 teaspoon ground cumin

3/4 teaspoon sea salt

1/2 teaspoon smoked paprika, preferably pimentón de la Vera

Soak the chickpeas overnight in enough water to cover by at least 2 inches. Drain and rinse.

Bring 1 cup water to a boil in an enameled cast iron paella pan or large skillet. Add the chickpeas, cover, and cook over medium-low heat for 22 to 25 minutes, until the chickpeas are tender but still slightly chewy.

Uncover, raise the heat to medium, and continue to cook, shaking and stirring the pan to roll them around for about 2 minutes longer, or until they are dry. Drizzle the olive oil over the chickpeas and stir to coat lightly.

Sprinkle on the cumin, salt, and smoked paprika. Cook, stirring, for 1 to 2 minutes longer to toast the spices. Serve warm or at room temperature.

# Thai Spring Rolls
### Makes 18 pieces; serves 4 to 6

This unconventional version of the classic Thai roll leaves off the rice noodles inside for a superlight bite of shrimp and vegetables. For those who've never used rice wrapping papers, they can be found in Asian groceries and some supermarkets. They are shelf stable and need no refrigeration. To use, simply dip briefly in water as directed below. They will continue to soften as they stand.

Thai Dipping Sauce (recipe follows)

$1/2$ pound peeled and deveined shrimp, fresh if you can get them or thawed if frozen

1 long, narrow seedless cucumber

2 medium carrots

12 round rice paper wrappers

2 scallions, minced

1 (4-ounce) package pea shoots

1 cup loosely packed cilantro sprigs

Prepare the dipping sauce. If you refrigerate it, return to room temperature before serving.

Bring a small pot of water to a boil. Add the shrimp and cook for about 3 minutes, until pink and curled. Drain and place in a bowl of ice water to cool and firm up for about 5 minutes. Drain again and blot dry. Cut lengthwise in half.

Peel the cucumber. Remove any seeds and cut the cucumber into thin, narrow strips about 5 inches long. Peel the carrots and cut them the same way.

To assemble the spring rolls, one at a time, dip a rice paper wrapper into a bowl of cold water for 10 to 20 seconds to soften. Carefully lay it down flat on a work surface. Dip a second wrapper and place it on top. Arrange 4 or 5 pieces of shrimp down the center of the wrappers. Sprinkle $1^1/_2$ to 2 teaspoons scallion over the shrimp. Add one-sixth of the cucumber and carrot. Using one-sixth of the package, arrange half the pea shoots facing one way and half the other, with the stem ends in the center and some of the leaves peaking out at the sides. Top generously with cilantro sprigs. Roll the rice papers up over the filling as snugly as possible without tearing; the ends will be open.

To serve, cut the rolls into thirds; there will be two pretty pieces, which should be set down with the pea shoots standing up. The third piece can stand up or lie on its side. Serve with the dipping sauce.

## THAI DIPPING SAUCE

Makes about $1/3$ cup

2 teaspoons brown sugar

$1/4$ cup warm water

2 tablespoons Thai or Vietnamese fish sauce

1 tablespoon freshly squeezed lime juice

2 teaspoons rice vinegar

$1/2$ small carrot, peeled and grated

1 small clove garlic, finely minced

In a small bowl, dissolve the brown sugar in the warm water. Add the fish sauce, lime juice, vinegar, carrot, and garlic, and stir to mix. If not using immediately, set aside at room temperature for up to 2 hours, or cover and refrigerate for up to 6 hours.

# Dilled Salmon Party Spread

Make about 1$^1$/$_2$ cups; serves 6 to 8

I call this a party spread because it's so good, you'll want to offer it to guests. Both fresh and smoked salmon are blended with light whipped cream cheese in place of butter, which can be difficult for GERD sufferers to digest. Either spread over the thick ends of Belgian endive spears or serve with whole-grain crackers.

6 ounces center-cut salmon fillet

Salt and freshly ground black pepper

1$^1$/$_2$ teaspoons extra virgin olive oil

3 ounces smoked salmon

4 ounces ($^1$/$_2$ cup) light whipped cream cheese

3 tablespoons chopped fresh dill

2 tablespoons minced fresh chives

Season the salmon with salt and pepper. Drizzle the olive oil over the meaty side. Grill the fish skin side up over a hot fire or in a grill pan for 2 minutes. Turn over and grill for 2 to 3 minutes, until just opaque in the center but still moist. Remove and let cool slightly, then discard the skin and trim off any dark brown bits along the center.

In a food processor, combine the grilled salmon, smoked salmon, cream cheese, dill, and chives. Season generously with pepper. Puree until blended to a spread. Serve at once or refrigerate for up to 3 days.

NOTE: For a larger party, the recipe doubles easily.

*Clockwise from top: Savory Goat Cheese Spread (page 75), Dilled Salmon Party Spread, and Romesco Sauce (page 74).*

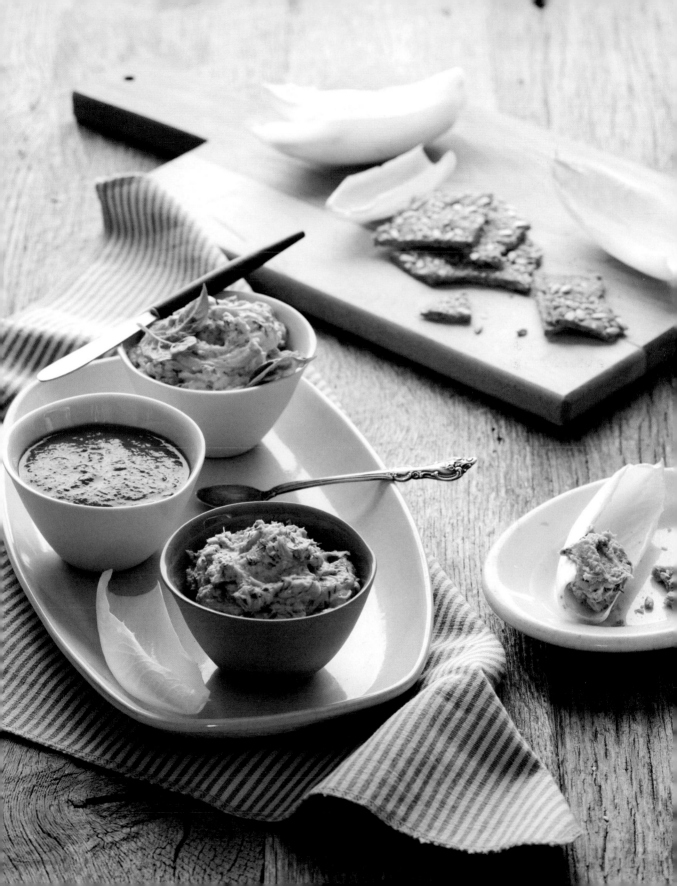

# Endive Spears with Tuna-Pistachio Tapenade
## Serves 6 to 8

Here's an easy, do-ahead hors d'oeuvre that takes just minutes. A fruity, rich-tasting extra virgin olive oil from Spain or Italy will make a big difference in this recipe, because the dish is so simple. If you can find both red and white endive, a mixture of the two looks very nice. Of course, the savory tuna mixture can be spread on crackers, sandwiched between a couple of slices of whole-grain bread, or scooped on top of a lovely salad.

1 (5-ounce) can light tuna packed in water or olive oil, well drained

3 tablespoons fruity extra virgin olive oil

1 1/2 teaspoons freshly squeezed lemon juice

1/4 cup pitted kalamata olives, chopped

1/4 cup shelled and roasted pistachio nuts, chopped

1 tablespoon minced fresh chives or dill

2 or 3 heads Belgian endive

In a small food processor, combine the tuna, olive oil, and lemon juice. Pulse until well blended.

Add the olives, pistachio nuts, and chives. Pulse until the olives and nuts are finely chopped. (The tuna tapenade can be made in advance and refrigerated for up to 24 hours.)

Rinse the endive and separate into about 24 large leaves. Spoon a heaping teaspoon of the tapendade onto the base of each leaf. Arrange attractively on a platter; a sunburst design is nice—a circle with the tips of the leaves facing outward. If not serving immediately, cover and refrigerate for up to 2 hours.

# Light and Lean Guacamole

Makes about 1$^1$/$_2$ cups; serves 4 to 6

Because avocados used to cost a small fortune—and are still not cheap in many parts of the country—it's not uncommon to use peas to stretch the expensive ingredient further. I used to think the idea was a little tacky, but that was before I did the math on calories and fat (even if it is so-called good fat). One cup of guacamole made with just avocado contains 481 calories; made with my combination of avocado and peas, 1 cup contains 200 calories. Who cares what's in it as long as the dip tastes good and you can indulge a little without counting every bite? That's assuming you use vegetable dunkers, of course: carrot sticks, cucumber slices, briefly steamed asparagus tips, or cauliflower or broccoli florets.

$^3$/$_4$ cup frozen baby peas

1 large or 2 small ripe avocados

1 to 1$^1$/$_2$ tablespoons freshly squeezed lemon juice

1 scallion, white and tender green parts,
    thinly sliced

1 small clove garlic, crushed through a press

$^1$/$_4$ to $^1$/$_2$ teaspoon sea salt

$^3$/$_4$ cup loosely packed cilantro sprigs

Steam the peas over boiling water for about 4 minutes, until they are tender but still bright green. Rinse under cold running water; drain well.

Place the peas in a food processor and puree until as smooth as possible. Scoop out and add the avocado, then add the lemon juice, scallion, garlic, and salt. Puree, stopping to scrape down the side of the bowl once or twice, until the dip is almost whipped.

Add the cilantro and pulse until chopped.

# Romesco Sauce

Makes about 1¼ cups; serves 6 to 8 as a dip

If you've never tasted this wonderful Basque sauce, you're in for a treat. Rich and smoky, it makes a marvelous dip for all kinds of vegetables. I like a mix of raw and lightly cooked vegetables. Contrary to what you often see, most vegetables enjoy better color and flavor—as well as contribute more of their vitamin content—when they are steamed for just a couple of minutes. Don't overdo it—just enough to set the color and soften them ever so slightly. But Romesco sauce is more than just a dip. It also makes a fabulous accompaniment to enliven simply cooked lamb, chicken, or fish. (Pictured on page 71.)

1 cup piquillo peppers or peeled, roasted red bell peppers (see note)

¼ cup sliced almonds, toasted (see note)

1 tablespoon freshly squeezed lemon juice

1 clove garlic, thinly sliced

¾ teaspoon smoked paprika, preferably pimentón de la Vera

½ teaspoon ground cumin

½ teaspoon salt

3 tablespoons cold water

2 tablespoons extra virgin olive oil

In a food processor, combine the peppers, almonds, lemon juice, garlic, paprika, cumin, and salt.

With the machine on, drizzle in the water and olive oil through the feed tube. Use at once or cover and refrigerate for up to 3 days.

NOTE: Piquillo peppers come in jars and offer a nice piquant but not hot note. Otherwise, ordinary peeled, roasted red bell peppers, which are available both jarred and in olive bars in many supermarkets, would do nicely.

I buy my almonds toasted and sliced, but if you want to toast your own raw almonds, toast them in a 325°F oven for about 7 minutes, or until fragrant and lightly browned.

# Savory Goat Cheese Spread

Makes about 1 cup

Saturated fat often takes the hardest toll on those with acid reflux. But avoiding it entirely is easier said than done. In general, goat cheese has less fat (and fewer calories) than cow's milk cheese. Here, the fresh white kind that comes in a narrow log is blended with light whipped cream cheese to cut the fat a little bit more. Enlivened with olives, rosemary, and just a hint of sun-dried tomatoes, this spread is great inside celery sticks or on whole-grain toast or crackers. (Pictured on page 71.)

6 ounces soft white goat cheese (chèvre), at
    room temperature

1/2 cup light whipped cream cheese

1 tablespoon extra virgin olive oil

1 small clove garlic, crushed

1/2 teaspoon coarsely cracked black pepper

1/4 cup pitted kalamata olives

2 tablespoons finely diced oil-packed sun-dried
    tomatoes

1 tablespoon finely chopped fresh basil, or
    1 1/2 teaspoons minced fresh rosemary
    (optional)

In a food processor, combine the goat cheese, cream cheese, olive oil, garlic, and pepper. Whirl until the mixture is evenly blended.

Add the olives and pulse until they are chopped. Transfer to a bowl and stir in the sun-dried tomatoes and basil.

Cover and refrigerate for at least 1 to 2 hours to chill and allow the flavors to mellow.

# Mushroom Polenta Tart

## Serves 8

Polenta, the Italian word for cornmeal, makes a great base in place of a traditional crust because it requires no fat. Here, it's topped with a savory wild mushroom ragout. Serve in small wedges as a first course, or form in a rectangular pan and cut into squares to pass as an hors d'oeuvre.

Salt and freshly ground black pepper

3/4 cup instant polenta

1 ounce (1/2 cup) dried porcini mushrooms

1 large shallot, minced

3 tablespoons extra virgin olive oil

1 pound baby bella or white mushrooms, sliced

1/4 pound fresh shiitakes, stemmed and sliced

1 teaspoon dried thyme

3/4 cup Easy Rotisserie Chicken Stock (page 87),
    or any reduced-sodium chicken broth

3/4 cup shredded provolone cheese

2 tablespoons chopped fresh parsley

Coat a 9½-inch tart pan with cooking spray. Bring 2 cups water to a boil with 1 teaspoon salt and ¼ teaspoon pepper in a heavy medium saucepan. Gradually sprinkle the polenta over the water while stirring until it is all incorporated. Reduce the heat to medium and cook, stirring, for about 5 minutes, until the polenta forms a mass and begins to pull away from the sides of the pan. Immediately spread out the hot polenta in the prepared tart pan. It will set as it cools.

In a small bowl, cover the porcini with boiling water and soak for 20 to 30 minutes, until softened. Lift them up, squeezing any extra liquid back into the bowl. Coarsely chop the mushrooms. Reserve ½ cup of the liquid, straining it through a coffee filter to remove any grit.

Meanwhile, in a large skillet, sauté the shallot in the olive oil over medium-high heat for 1 minute. Add the bella mushrooms and sauté, stirring often, for 5 to 7 minutes, until they are lightly browned. Add the shiitakes, chopped porcini, and thyme. Season liberally with salt and pepper.

Pour in the stock and the porcini soaking liquid. Bring to a boil, partially cover, and simmer for about 15 minutes, until the liquid is absorbed. Spread the mushroom ragout over the polenta crust. Scatter the cheese over the top. The recipe can be prepared ahead to this point and set aside at room temperature for up to 5 hours or refrigerated for up to 8 hours.

Shortly before serving, preheat the oven to 400°F. Bake the tart for 10 to 15 minutes, until the cheese melts and the polenta is heated through. Sprinkle with the parsley before serving.

# Thin-Crust Pizza with Spinach and Goat Cheese

Serves 4 as a light main course, or 6 as a starter

No one wants to give up pizza, even if they do suffer from reflux. Here's a solution: a very thin crust made light and tender with mashed potatoes. Where a pound of pizza flour would normally make one large pizza, this recipes makes two. Less flour and smaller portions should keep you in the clear. Cut into small pieces, it makes an ever-popular pick-up hors d'oeuvre. If you'd rather serve it for supper, this recipe allows two generous slices of pizza per person.

1/2 recipe Mashed Potato Pizza Dough (recipe follows)

1 small onion, chopped

3 1/2 tablespoons extra virgin olive oil

1 or 2 cloves garlic, thinly sliced

1 teaspoon minced fresh rosemary, or 1/2 teaspoon crumbled dried

1/2 teaspoon Aleppo pepper (optional; see note)

2 1/2 to 3 ounces shredded part-skim mozzarella cheese (3/4 cup)

3 to 4 ounces baby spinach

2 1/2 ounces soft white goat cheese (chèvre)

Coat an 18-inch perforated pizza pan or an 8 by 12-inch rimmed baking sheet with cooking spray.

Make the pizza dough as directed.

While the dough is resting, in a medium skillet, cook the onion in 2 tablespoons of the olive oil over medium-high heat for 5 to 7 minutes, until golden. Add the garlic and cook for 1 minute longer. Remove from the heat and set aside.

Preheat the oven to 450°F. Roll or press the dough out to cover the prepared pan. Scrape the golden onions with the olive oil and garlic over the dough and spread out evenly with your fingertips. Sprinkle the rosemary and Aleppo pepper over the dough. Bake for 8 to 10 minutes, until the dough is dry on top.

Sprinkle the mozzarella over the pizza. Top with the spinach and dot with the goat cheese. Drizzle the remaining 1 1/2 tablespoons olive oil over the pizza. Bake for 8 to 10 minutes longer, until the crust is crisp.

NOTE: Aleppo pepper is a wonderful mildly hot pepper with good flavor, which makes a nice stand-in for the spicer varieties. If you think you cannot tolerate any heat at all, substitute freshly ground black peppercorns.

*Continued*

## MASHED POTATO PIZZA DOUGH

Makes enough for 2 pizzas

1 large baking potato, 10 to 12 ounces, peeled and
    cut into 1-inch chunks

Salt

1 pound refrigerated pizza dough (not whole wheat;
    see note)

Place the potato chunks in a small saucepan and add enough salted water to cover by 1 inch. Bring to a boil over high heat and cook for 10 to 12 minutes, until soft. Drain and put the potato through a ricer or mash with a potato masher or fork until smooth. Let cool slightly.

With your fingers, work the mashed potato into the pizza dough until evenly blended. Knead into a ball, place in an oiled bowl, cover with plastic wrap, and let stand at room temperature for 20 minutes. Divide the dough in half. If making only 1 pizza, the remaining dough can be wrapped and refrigerated overnight, or frozen for up to 2 months.

NOTE: While more fiber is generally recommended, I find whole wheat pizza and pasta difficult to digest. It's just too heavy and forms an exception to the rule.

# SOUPS

# Butternut Squash and Pear Bisque

### Serves 6 to 8

Soups are a little tricky when you have GERD. On the one hand, they are light in texture, sometimes high in fiber, relatively low in fat, and very economical calorie-wise. But since we're emphasizing low volume as a major component of the Acid Reflux Solution, soup cannot be a "free food." This lush squash bisque, lightly sweetened with pear and just a touch of maple syrup, makes a delightful starter or companion to half a sandwich or a salad for lunch.

1 butternut squash, preferably organic (about 1¹/2 pounds)

1 medium leek, white and tender green parts, sliced

2 tablespoons extra virgin olive oil

1 ripe Barlett pear, peeled, cored, and cut into 1-inch chunks

1 teaspoon sea salt

1 teaspoon winter savory or thyme

¹/4 teaspoon freshly grated nutmeg

6 cups Easy Rotisserie Chicken Stock (page 87), or any reduced-sodium chicken broth

¹/4 cup heavy cream

1 tablespoon maple syrup

Preheat the oven to 400°F. Split the squash lengthwise in half. Set cut sides down in a lightly oiled pie plate or baking dish and roast for 35 to 45 minutes, until tender. With a large spoon, scoop out the seeds and membranes. Peel off the outer skin. Cut the squash into 1¹/2-inch chunks.

In a large enameled flameproof casserole or stainless steel saucepan, cook the leek in the olive oil over medium heat, stirring occasionally, for about 5 minutes, until softened. Add the squash, pear, salt, savory, and nutmeg. Pour in the stock and bring to a boil. Reduce the heat to medium-low, partially cover, and simmer for 20 minutes. Stir in the cream.

Puree the soup right in the pot with an immersion blender or transfer to a food processor or blender in batches and puree until smooth. Reheat the soup. Whisk in the maple syrup and simmer, uncovered, for 5 minutes. Serve hot.

# Carrot Bisque with Ginger Cream

### Serves 6

Aromatic with spices and softened with a ginger yogurt cream, this smooth soup goes down easily. Enjoy a small cup, followed by a salad.

1/2 yellow onion, finely chopped

2 1/2 tablespoons extra virgin olive oil

2 tablespoons unbleached all-purpose flour

1 tablespoon ground coriander

2 teaspoons ground cumin

6 cups Easy Rotisserie Chicken Stock (page 87), or any reduced-sodium chicken broth

1/2 pound carrots, peeled and sliced

1 tablespoon minced fresh ginger

2 teaspoons demerara or turbinado sugar

1 cup plain low-fat Greek-style yogurt

In a large stainless steel saucepan or enameled flameproof casserole, cook the onion in the olive oil over medium heat for 5 to 7 minutes, until soft and golden. Sprinkle on the flour, coriander, and cumin. Cook, stirring often, for 1 to 2 minutes, to toast without coloring.

Whisk in the stock and bring to a boil, whisking until thickened and smooth. Add the carrots, reduce the heat to a simmer, and partially cover. Cook for about 20 minutes, or until the carrots are very tender. Use an immersion blender to puree the soup in the pot or transfer to a food processor or blender, in batches if necessary, and puree until smooth; return to the pot.

Whisk the ginger and sugar into the yogurt. Whisk 2/3 cup of the ginger cream into the soup. Ladle into bowls. Top each with a dollop of the remaining cream.

# Chunky Beet Soup with Ginger and Orange

Serves 6 to 8

Orange, ginger, and beets make a fabulous flavor combination. While a glass of orange juice is highly acidic and likely to cause reflux, the small amount of fresh juice in this soup will not trigger anything but the desire for more. Serve this gorgeous soup plain or with a dollop of yogurt and sprinkling of chives.

1 yellow onion, diced

3 tablespoons extra virgin olive oil

2 cups diced green cabbage (about 8 ounces)

2 teaspoons ground coriander

1 teaspoon dried thyme leaves, preferably lemon thyme

$1/8$ teaspoon ground cloves

1 bay leaf

1 pound raw beets, peeled and diced

6 cups Easy Rotisserie Chicken Stock (page 87), or any reduced-sodium chicken broth

2 large carrots, peeled and sliced or diced

2 tablespoons chopped fresh parsley

2 teaspoons grated fresh ginger

Grated zest and juice from $1/2$ orange

Sea salt and freshly ground black pepper

In a large stainless steel saucepan or enameled flameproof casserole, cook the onion in the olive oil over medium-low heat, covered, for about 3 minutes, until soft. Then uncover, raise the heat to medium-high, and sauté for 3 to 5 minutes, until the onion begins to brown.

Add the cabbage and continue to cook, stirring occasionally, for about 5 minutes longer, until the cabbage is wilted and just starts to color. Add the coriander, thyme, cloves, and bay leaf. Cook for 2 minutes, stirring often.

Reduce the heat to medium-low. Add the beets and the stock. Bring to a boil slowly, partially covered, taking 10 to 15 minutes. Add the carrots, raise the heat to medium, and continue to cook for 10 to 15 minutes longer, until the vegetables are tender.

Add the parsley, ginger, and orange zest. Simmer for 10 minutes. Remove from the heat and stir in the orange juice. Season with salt and pepper to taste. Discard the bay leaf. Serve hot or chilled.

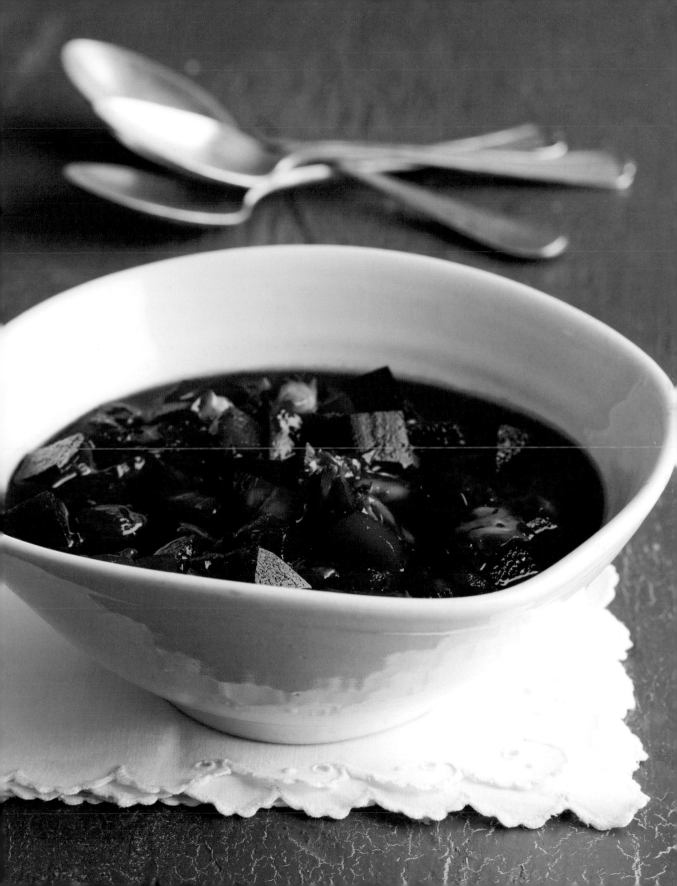

# Cauliflower and Watercress Soup

Serves 6

Easy on the tummy and exceptionally nutritious, this is a vegetable soup you can enjoy any time of the year. While watercress has a little bit of a bite that might scare some, cooking it for even a few minutes tames the sharpness completely. Arugula or spinach can substitute for the cress.

1 small leek, white and tender green parts, sliced

2 tablespoons unsalted butter

1 tablespoon olive oil

3 tablespoons unbleached all-purpose flour

6 cups Easy Rotisserie Chicken Stock (page 87), or any reduced-sodium chicken broth

1 head cauliflower (1 to 1½ pounds), separated into florets

1 large bunch watercress, cut into 1-inch lengths, tough stems discarded

Salt and freshly ground black pepper

In a large stainless steel saucepan or enameled flameproof casserole, cook the leek in the butter and oil over medium heat for 3 to 5 minutes, until softened.

Sprinkle on the flour and cook, stirring often, for 2 minutes. Whisk in the stock and bring to a boil, whisking until the liquid is smooth and slightly thickened.

Add the cauliflower. Bring to a boil, reduce the heat, and partially cover. Cook for about 15 minutes, until the cauliflower is soft. Add the watercress and cook for 3 to 5 minutes longer, until the stems are tender but the leaves are still bright green.

Use an immersion blender to puree the soup in the pot or transfer to a food processor or blender, in batches if necessary, and puree until smooth; return to the pot. Season with salt and pepper to taste. Rewarm before serving.

# Chilled Avocado and Cucumber Soup

Serves 6 to 8

Many people with GERD think they cannot tolerate cucumbers, but the long, narrow seedless English and baby Persian varieties with very thin skins are much more digestible in general. Pureeing them like this with silky avocado produces an elixir that goes down easily and hopefully will not bother you at all.

2 ripe avocados

3 small Persian cucumbers, or ½ long, narrow
    seedless cucumber

⅓ cup fresh dill sprigs, plus extra for garnish

1 small shallot, thinly sliced

4 cups Easy Rotisserie Chicken Stock (page 87),
    any reduced-sodium chicken broth, or
    vegetable broth

1 cup plain yogurt

Salt and freshly ground black pepper

Halve the avocados, remove the pits, and scoop the flesh into a food processor or blender.

Depending upon your sensitivity, completely peel the cucumbers or remove just half the peel. Cut lengthwise in half and scoop out any seeds. Cut the cucumbers into chunks and add to the avocado along with the dill, shallot, and 1 cup of the stock. Puree until smooth.

With the machine on, gradually add the remaining 3 cups stock and ⅔ cup of the yogurt. Season with salt and pepper to taste. Cover and refrigerate for about 2 hours, until thoroughly chilled. Ladle into soup plates. Garnish each serving with a small dollop of the remaining ⅓ cup yogurt and a dill sprig.

# Cuban Black Bean Soup
Serves 6 to 8

Here's a quick and easy version of one of my favorite recipes. Because it is filling, I suggest it for lunch, topped with a dollop of plain yogurt and accompanied by a nice avocado salad, such as Arugula and Avocado Salad with Blueberries and Melon (page 97).

1 yellow onion, chopped

3 tablespoons extra virgin olive oil

2 celery ribs, chopped

2 carrots, peeled and chopped

1/2 green bell pepper, seeded and chopped

1 1/2 teaspoons cumin seed, crushed

1 teaspoon dried oregano

2 (16-ounce) cans black beans, preferably organic, rinsed and drained

4 cups Easy Rotisserie Chicken Stock (page 87), or any reduced-sodium chicken broth

1 bay leaf

1 tablespoon sherry wine vinegar

Salt and freshly ground black pepper

Plain low-fat yogurt (optional)

In a large saucepan or enameled flameproof casserole, cook the onion in the olive oil over medium heat for about 5 minutes, until softened and beginning to turn golden. Add the celery, carrot, and bell pepper and cook for 3 to 5 minutes, until the celery is soft. Stir in the cumin seed and oregano and cook for 2 minutes longer.

Add the black beans, stock, and bay leaf. Bring to a boil, reduce the heat, and simmer, partially covered, for 20 minutes. Remove and discard the bay leaf.

Either use an immersion blender to partially puree the soup or transfer 2 cups to a food processor or blender, puree until smooth, and return to the remaining soup. Stir in the vinegar. Season with salt and pepper to taste. Serve hot, with a dollop of yogurt on top, if you like.

# Easy Rotisserie Chicken Stock

Makes 4 to 6 cups

How many times have you purchased a rotisserie chicken and thrown away the bones? No more. Save the carcass, bones, and skin to make this lovely simple stock.

1 whole clove

1 yellow onion, halved

Carcass and bones from 1 rotisserie chicken

2 cloves garlic, halved

1 bay leaf

1/2 teaspoon dried thyme leaves

1/2 teaspoon black peppercorns

Stick the clove into the onion. Put the onion and chicken carcass and bones in a large saucepan. Add enough water to almost fill the pot. Bring to a boil, skimming off any foam that rises to the top.

Add the garlic, bay leaf, thyme, and peppercorns. Reduce the heat to low and simmer, uncovered, for 2 to 3 hours. If too much water evaporates, add more so that you end up with 1 to 1 1/2 quarts of stock. Remove and discard the bay leaf.

Let cool, then remove any fat that forms on top. Cover and refrigerate for up to 3 days or freeze for up to 2 months.

# Scallop-Corn Chowder

### Serves 4 to 6

How amazing that a chowder this good contains no milk. If you don't tell, I'd be surprised if anyone will guess the light but rich-tasting base is soy. Serve this lovely chowder garnished with a sprinkling of chopped chervil or chives.

1 small leek, white and tender green parts

2 tablespoons unsalted butter or extra virgin olive oil

2 1/2 tablespoons unbleached all-purpose flour

2 teaspoons vegetable bouillon powder dissolved in 2 cups boiling water

1 1/2 cups diced Yukon gold potatoes (about 1 1/4 pounds)

1/2 teaspoon dried lemon thyme leaves

1/8 teaspoon freshly grated nutmeg

1 2/3 cups plain enriched organic soy milk (see note)

1/3 cup heavy cream

1 1/2 cups fresh or canned corn

1/2 pound small bay scallops, or sea scallops cut into 1/2-inch dice

Salt and freshly ground black pepper

Cut the leek in half lengthwise, then thinly slice. Place in a small bowl of water and swish around to remove any sand. Remove and drain.

In a 4-quart flameproof casserole or large saucepan, melt the butter. Add the leek to the pot. Cook over medium-low heat for about 3 minutes, until softened. Sprinkle on the flour and cook, stirring, for 1 to 2 minutes longer, to cook without coloring.

Pour in the dissolved bouillon water and bring to a boil, stirring and scraping the bottom of the pot, until the liquid is thickened and smooth. Add the potatoes and season with the thyme and nutmeg. Partially cover and boil gently for 12 to 15 minutes, until the potatoes are just tender.

Pour in the soy milk and cream and bring to a boil, stirring until the soup thickens slightly. Add the corn and scallops, reduce the heat, and simmer for 5 minutes longer. Season with salt and pepper to taste. Serve hot.

NOTE: For best flavor, choose a neutral soy milk that does not have added sugar or vanilla flavoring, such as organic Eden brand.

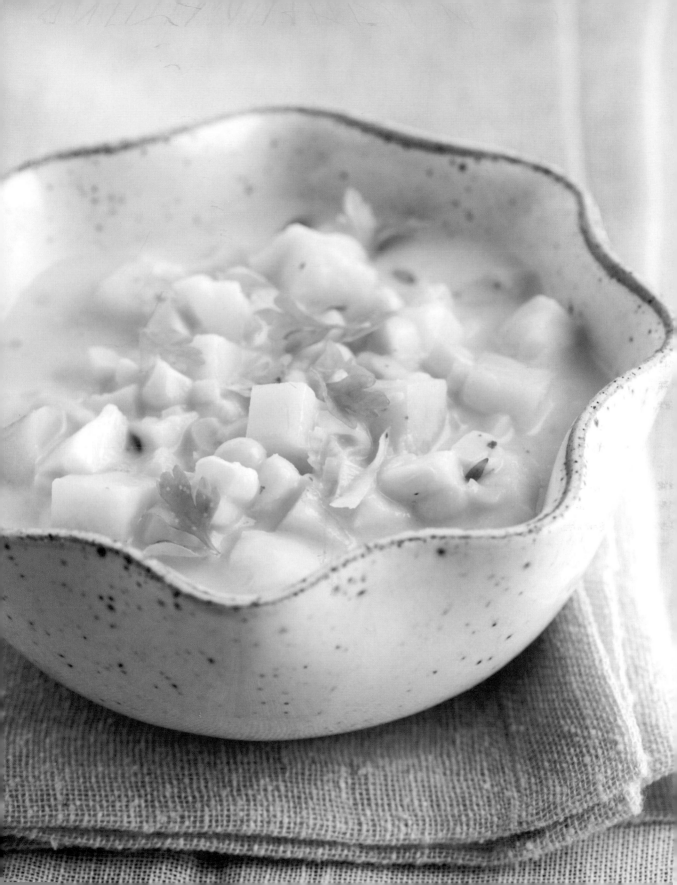

# Garden Vegetable Soup

## Serves 6

Here's supper in a bowl, and plenty of healthy fiber. Accompany with a slice of whole-grain bread, grilled with a slice of tangy cheese on top, like Manchego or Midnight Moon. Yes, there are tomatoes in this soup, but they are quite diluted, and if you stick to $1^1/_2$ cups as a serving and resist seconds, you should have no problem at all. Like so many dishes that contain cabbage and tomato, this soup tastes even better when reheated.

1 small yellow onion, diced

3 tablespoons extra virgin olive oil

$^3/_4$ pound green cabbage, cut into $^1/_2$-inch dice

2 medium Yukon gold or red-skinned potatoes, peeled and cut into $^1/_2$-inch dice

2 medium-large carrots, peeled and cut into about $^1/_2$-inch dice

2 cups vegetable stock, Easy Rotisserie Chicken Stock (page 87), or any reduced-sodium chicken broth

3 large Roma tomatoes, peeled, seeded, and diced

2 ounces green beans, cut into $^1/_2$-inch pieces ($^3/_4$ cup)

$1^1/_2$ cups fresh or canned corn

$^1/_2$ cup frozen baby peas

Sea salt and freshly ground black pepper

In a large soup pot, cook the onion in the olive oil over medium heat, covered, for 3 minutes, until soft. Uncover, raise the heat to medium-high, and cook for about 2 minutes longer, until the onion just starts to color.

Add the cabbage, potatoes, and carrots. Pour in the stock, tomatoes, and 4 cups water. Bring to a boil over high heat, reduce the heat slightly, and boil, partially covered, for 7 minutes.

Add the green beans, corn, and peas and cook for 5 to 7 minutes longer, until the beans are tender. Season with salt and pepper to taste. Serve hot.

# Fennel-Scented Lentil Soup

## Serves 6

Lentil soup comes in many forms, from a stick-to-your ribs porridge to spicy Indian mulligatawny. This subtly flavored version, light enough to sip from a cup, is fragrant with fresh fennel and fennel seed. Offer it as a first course or enjoy a mugful in between meals as a low-calorie snack with healthy fiber.

1 yellow onion, chopped

3 tablespoons sunflower or extra virgin olive oil

1 celery rib, chopped

1/2 fresh fennel bulb, with some fronds, chopped

1/3 green bell pepper, seeded and chopped

2 medium-large carrots, chopped

1 cup lentils, preferably the tiny green French lentilles du Puy

1 tablespoon vegetable bouillon powder (optional but nice)

1/2 teaspoon crushed fennel seed

1 bay leaf

Salt and freshly ground black pepper

In a large flameproof casserole, sauté the onion in the oil over medium-high heat for about 5 minutes, until golden. Add the celery, fennel, and bell pepper. Sauté for 5 minutes longer, or until the celery and fennel are softened.

Add the carrots, lentils, and 8 cups water. Bring to a boil. Stir in the bouillon powder and add the fennel seed and bay leaf. Reduce the heat to medium-low, partially cover, and simmer for 30 to 35 minutes, until the lentils are just tender. Remove and discard the bay leaf.

Using an immersion blender, partially puree the soup, leaving about half the lentils intact. Or transfer about 3 cups of the soup to a food processor or blender and puree until smooth; return the soup to the pot. Simmer uncovered for 20 minutes.

Season with salt and pepper to taste. Serve hot.

# Mushroom Bisque with Tarragon and Chives

### Serves 4 to 6

Too much liquid can add pressure to the abdomen the same way that too much food can. That's why just a small cup of this intense, elegant soup is the perfect way to start a meal.

1 pound white mushrooms

1/4 pound fresh shiitakes

1 small leek, white and tender green parts, thinly sliced

4 cups Easy Rotisserie Chicken Stock (page 87), or any reduced-sodium chicken broth

1 teaspoon freshly squeezed lemon juice

1 teaspoon dried tarragon

2 tablespoons unsalted butter

2 1/2 tablespoons unbleached all-purpose flour

1 cup plain enriched organic soy milk (see note)

Salt and freshly ground black pepper

Minced fresh chives

Trim the stem ends and quarter 3/4 pound of the white mushrooms. Thinly slice the remainder. Remove and discard the shiitake stems. Slice the caps and set aside.

In a food processor, pulse the quartered mushrooms until coarsely chopped. Transfer to a 2- to 3-quart saucepan. Add the leek, stock, lemon juice, and tarragon. Bring to a simmer over medium-high heat, partially cover, and reduce the heat. Simmer for 15 minutes. Strain through a fine-mesh sieve set over a bowl, pressing down on the mushrooms and leeks with a wooden spoon to extract as much liquid as possible. Discard the contents of the sieve.

In a heavy pot, melt the butter over medium heat. Add the flour and cook, stirring, for 1 to 2 minutes, without browning. Whisk in 2 cups of the hot mushroom stock and bring to a boil, whisking until thickened and smooth. Whisk in the remaining stock and return to a boil. Add the soy milk and season with salt and pepper to taste.

Bring to a bare simmer and add the sliced white and shiitake mushrooms. Simmer for 5 to 10 minutes, until just tender. Ladle the bisque into small soup bowls and garnish each serving with a sprinkling of minced chives.

NOTE: For best flavor, choose a neutral soy milk that does not have added sugar or vanilla flavoring, such as organic Eden brand.

Chapter 9

# SALADS

# Arugula and Hearts of Palm Salad

Serves 4

Despite the fact that palm oil is heavily saturated, hearts of palm are virtually fat free. If you have a choice, buy the kind in a jar, because they can pick up a metallic taste from a tin. This elegant little salad makes a perfect starter. Depending upon your sensitivity scale, include ripe cherry tomatoes or opt for beets. Mâche, which is a milder green, can also be substituted for the arugula.

6 cups (about 6 ounces) baby arugula or mâche

2 1/2 tablespoons extra virgin olive oil

1 1/2 teaspoons walnut oil

2 teaspoons sherry wine vinegar

1 teaspoon freshly squeezed lemon juice

Salt and freshly ground black pepper

6 ounces hearts of palm, sliced

16 cherry tomatoes, halved, or 3/4 cup Balsamic Beets (page 165)

2 ounces feta cheese, crumbled

1/4 cup coarsely chopped walnuts or pecans, toasted (see note)

In a bowl, toss the arugula with the olive oil, walnut oil, vinegar, and lemon juice. Season lightly with salt and pepper. Divide the dressed greens among 4 salad plates.

Arrange the hearts of palm slices and cherry tomatoes decoratively on top. Sprinkle with the feta cheese and garnish with the chopped toasted nuts.

NOTE: To toast the nuts, preheat the oven to 325°F. Place the nuts in a single layer in a small baking dish and toast for 5 to 7 minutes, until fragrant and very lightly browned.

# Barley Salad with Corn and Edamame

## Serves 6

Texture plays a big part in the appeal of this simple salad, with the chewy grain playing off the firm edamame and almost crunchy corn. Serve with some tossed greens for a light vegetarian lunch, or offer as a side in place of potato salad. While this dish is full of fiber and very easy to digest, if you suspect you have an intolerance to wheat, keep in mind that barley does contain gluten.

1 cup pearl barley

1 tablespoon vegetable bouillon powder

1 cup fresh or frozen corn kernels

1 cup frozen edamame (shelled soybeans)

2 tablespoons extra virgin olive oil

1 tablespoon sherry wine vinegar or red or white wine vinegar

2 tablespoons coarsely chopped fresh dill

Salt and freshly ground black pepper

In a small saucepan, cook the barley in 2½ cups water with the bouillon powder for 20 to 25 minutes, until the barley is tender but still slightly chewy.

Meanwhile, steam the corn for 2 to 3 minutes, until just heated through. Steam the edamame for about 3 minutes, until hot and tender but still firm. Set the vegetables aside.

In a serving bowl, toss the barley with the olive oil, vinegar, 1½ tablespoons of the dill, and salt and pepper to taste. Add the corn and edamame and fold gently to mix. Sprinkle the remaining ½ tablespoon dill on top. Serve warm, at room temperature, or slightly chilled.

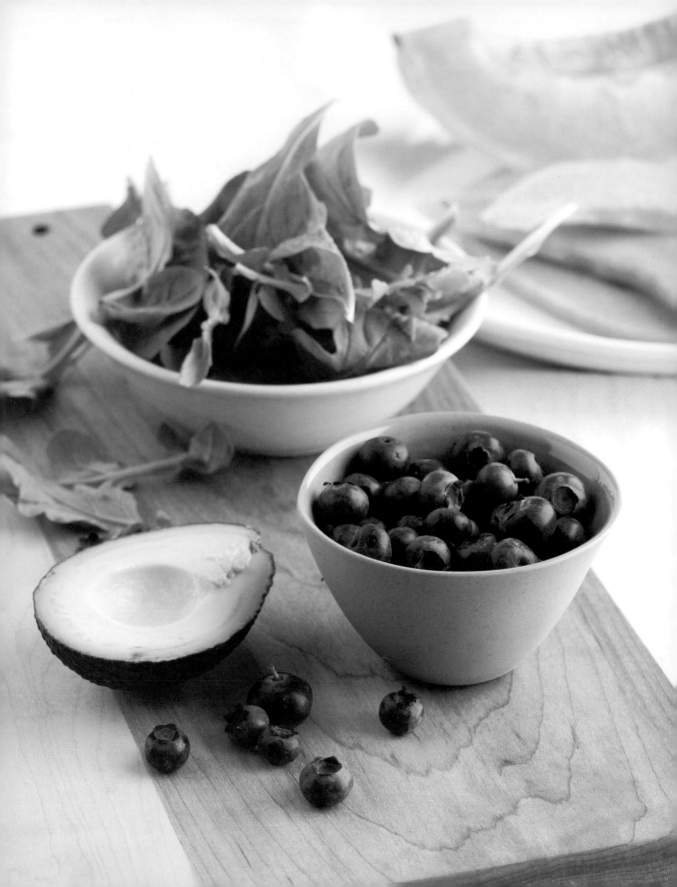

# Arugula and Avocado Salad with Blueberries and Melon

### Serves 1

Salad is almost always a good first choice for GERD sufferers. The plant fiber aids digestion and also fills you up with fewer calories, so that portion control is easier to maintain in the meal that follows. This is a really pretty salad that can easily be turned into a main-course lunch with a sprinkling of sunflower seeds and a few tablespoons of crumbled ricotta salata, white goat cheese, or feta.

1 cup arugula

2 (1-inch-wide) slices cantaloupe or honeydew, rind removed

$1/2$ small avocado, cut lengthwise into $1/2$-inch slices

$1/4$ cup blueberries

2 teaspoons freshly squeezed Meyer lemon juice, or $1 1/2$ teaspoons white wine vinegar

1 tablespoon extra virgin olive oil

Arrange the arugula on a plate. Decoratively arrange the melon and avocado slices on top. Scatter the blueberries over the salad.

Drizzle the lemon juice and olive oil over all and serve at once.

# Cool Cilantro Slaw

Serves 4

Many people don't realize it because the vegetable is so mild, but cabbage is packed with vitamin C, one of the most important antioxidants there is. It does double-duty, mopping up dangerous chemicals in your body and converting them into harmless substances, one of which is water, which can be excreted. If you've cut way down on citrus because of acid reflux, be sure you get your vitamin C elsewhere, such as in this simple slaw. It may seem odd not to include any mayonnaise or oil, but think of all the refreshing Thai and Indonesian salads that are entirely fat free. I like this as a side salad or to add flavor and texture to a turkey sandwich. For best texture, prepare shortly before serving. Compared to other vinegars, rice vinegar is very low in acid and in such a small amount, should not bother your stomach at all.

4 cups finely sliced green cabbage (about
     $1/3$ medium head cabbage)

1 teaspoon demerara or turbinado sugar

$1/2$ teaspoon salt

2 tablespoons rice vinegar diluted with
     1 tablespoon ice cold water

2 tablespoons freshly chopped cilantro

Toss the cabbage with the sugar and salt. Let stand for 5 minutes. Drizzle on the diluted vinegar. Add the cilantro, toss, and serve.

# Red and Green Ginger-Sesame Slaw

Serves 4

Ginger has long been believed to have healing properties for the stomach. Sailors use it to combat nausea, and the Chinese tout it as a digestive aid. Here, glacéed ginger, which is candied, chewy, and sweet, adds lively interest to a simple but very pretty slaw that goes well with many grilled dishes and sandwiches. Rice vinegar has a much lower acidity than others. In such a small amount and diluted with water, it's almost undetectable.

3 cups shredded green cabbage

1 cup shredded red cabbage

2 tablespoons finely minced glacéed ginger

1 1/2 teaspoons finely minced fresh ginger

1/4 teaspoon sea salt

1 1/2 tablespoons rice vinegar diluted with
    1 tablespoon water

4 teaspoons toasted sesame oil

In a bowl, combine all the ingredients and toss well. Serve at once or let stand at room temperature for up to 1 hour. This slaw holds up well in the refrigerator for up to 24 hours.

# Greek Salad with Chickpeas and Feta Cheese

Serves 4

Raw green bell pepper, usually one of the hallmark ingredients of a Greek salad, has been omitted here, because while it is technically not a trigger food, it does tend to "repeat" on many people. I'm going out on a limb and including a small amount of onion, rinsed and marinated in the dressing first, which removes the bite. The same kind of insoluble fiber, called inulin, that makes onion somewhat indigestible has protective properties as well, so I think it's worth a try; but if you know it will bother you, simply leave it out.

Feta cheese can vary greatly in flavor, depending on where it is from and what type of milk it's made from. Because you want the most flavor ounce for ounce, I recommend Greek feta, which is made from sheep's milk and has a robust taste.

1 cup Chickpea Poppers (page 67), or canned chickpeas, rinsed and drained

1 head romaine lettuce

2 small Persian cucumbers, or $1/2$ long, narrow seedless cucumber

1 large red bell pepper

$1/3$ cup sliced white or red onion (optional)

1 tablespoon red wine vinegar

1 tablespoon freshly squeezed lemon juice

Salt and freshly ground black pepper

12 cherry tomatoes, halved (optional)

8 pitted kalamata olives, quartered lengthwise

2 tablespoons coarsely chopped fresh dill, or $3/4$ teaspoon dried oregano

3 ounces feta cheese, preferably Greek, diced

$1/4$ cup extra virgin olive oil

If you plan to top your salad with the chickpea poppers, you can make them first and store at room temperature until ready to use.

Trim the lettuce, separate into leaves, and rinse well. Cut or tear into large pieces; you want about 8 cups. Soak in a salad spinner or large bowl with a cup of ice cubes to crisp up while you prepare the rest of the salad.

Peel the cucumbers and cut into $1/2$-inch dice. Both these varieties are supposed to be seedless, but if you see any, scoop them out. Using a swivel-bladed vegetable peeler, peel the bell pepper. Cut into $1/2$-inch dice.

Cut the onion slices into thirds. Place in a strainer and rinse briefly under cold running water; drain well. Place in a large salad bowl and toss with the vinegar and lemon juice. Season generously with salt and pepper. Add the cucumbers, red pepper, tomatoes, olives, dill, feta, and 1 tablespoon of the olive oil. Toss

*Continued*

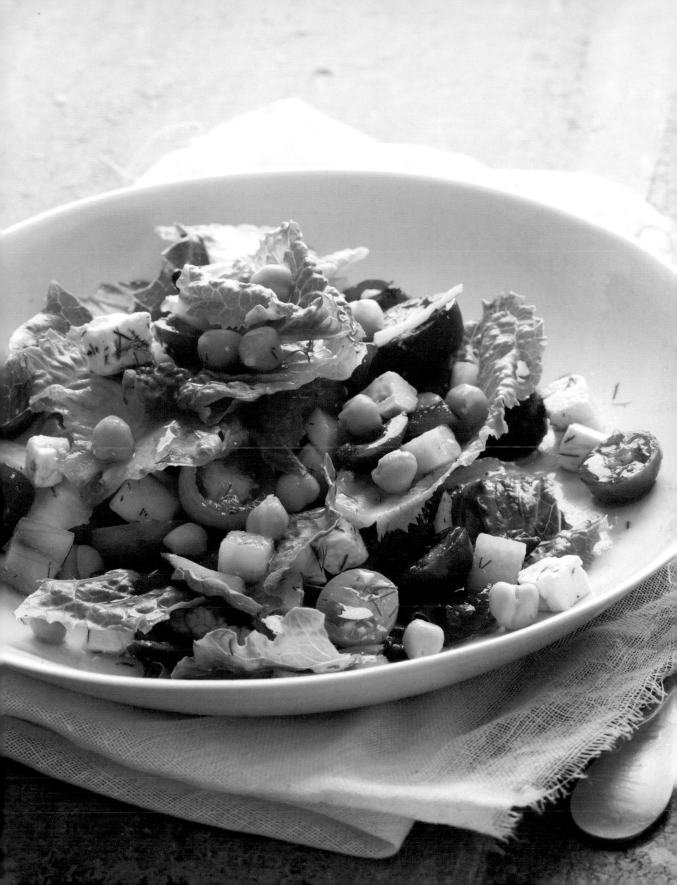

again gently and let stand for about 5 minutes, or until you finish preparing the rest of the ingredients.

Drain the romaine lettuce and spin dry. Add the lettuce to the rest of the salad. Top with the chickpeas. Drizzle on the remaining 3 tablespoons olive oil and toss to mix evenly.

NOTE: That there are no anchovies here has nothing to do with GERD. I love them, but none of my friends will touch them, so I'm used to leaving them out. If you like them, by all means arrange half a tin on top.

# Chopped Chef's Salad

Serves 4

Lunch is a great time to manage those calories and pack in a lot of fiber, but even here, you've got to watch your portions. I make a different salad almost every day. But by salad, I don't mean just lettuce. Any vegetable is fair game. Punch it up with small amounts of tasty cheese and lean meat, and don't skimp when you shop for oils and vinegars. They provide the base upon which all good salads are built.

$1/2$ cup diced fresh fennel or celery

$1/2$ cup diced cooked beets, Balsamic Beets (page 165), or red bell pepper

$1/2$ cup diced carrot

1 small Persian cucumber, diced

16 grape tomatoes, halved or quartered (optional)

Sea salt and freshly ground black pepper

1 tablespoon Banyuls or sherry wine vinegar

1 tablespoon walnut or extra virgin olive oil

4 ounces roast turkey, diced or cut into strips

2 ounces lean nitrate-free ham, such as Applegate uncured Black Forest ham, diced or cut into strips

2 ounces tasty firm cheese, such as Midnight Moon or an aged Cheddar, diced

6 cups torn romaine lettuce

2 tablespoons extra virgin olive oil

2 tablespoons sunflower seeds

In a large salad bowl, toss together the fennel, beets, carrot, cucumber, and tomatoes. Season with salt and pepper to taste. Sprinkle on the vinegar and walnut oil, toss, and let stand for a few minutes to marinate.

Add the turkey, ham, and cheese. Toss to mix.

Just before serving, add the lettuce, drizzle the olive oil over the salad, and toss again. Divide among 4 plates and sprinkle the sunflower seeds on top.

# Buffalo Chicken Salad with Blue Cheese and Light Ranch Dressing

### Serves 4

Blue cheese is definitely not low in fat, but it's so intensely flavored, all you need is a little bit. This tasty salad has all the good flavors of buffalo wings, minus the heat. For those who can deal with intense spice, pass a bottle of hot sauce on the side.

Light Ranch Dressing (recipe follows)

12 ounces skinless, boneless chicken breasts

1 cup buttermilk

2 tablespoons minced yellow onion

1 teaspoon thyme

Salt and freshly ground black pepper

3/4 cup panko bread crumbs

1 teaspoon smoked paprika, preferably pimentón de la Vera

1 small head iceberg lettuce, shredded (6 to 8 cups)

1 1/2 ounces Roquefort or other strong blue-veined cheese

Make the dressing and refrigerate until ready to use.

Trim any fat or gristle from the chicken breasts, open them up as much as you can, and pound lightly to flatten evenly to about 1/2 inch.

In a pie plate or shallow bowl, combine the buttermilk, onion, 1/2 teaspoon of the thyme, 1/2 teaspoon salt, and 1/8 teaspoon pepper. Add the chicken breasts and marinate at room temperature for 20 to 30 minutes.

Preheat the oven to 400°F. On a sheet of waxed paper or a large plate, toss the bread crumbs with the paprika, remaining 1/2 teaspoon thyme, 1/4 teaspoon salt, and a generous grind of pepper. Lift the chicken out of the marinade and dredge in the crumbs to coat. Set on an oiled baking sheet.

Bake the chicken breasts for 15 to 20 minutes, until they are just cooked through and white in the center and the crumb coating is golden. As soon as the chicken is cool enough to handle, use a sharp knife to cut the breasts crosswise into 1/2-inch-wide strips.

In a large bowl, toss the lettuce with the ranch dressing to coat. Divide among 4 plates. Arrange the chicken over the lettuce and crumble the cheese on top.

## LIGHT RANCH DRESSING

Makes about $1/2$ cup

Reduced-fat sour cream, low-fat buttermilk, and just enough mayonnaise to bind make this a marvelous "light" dressing. Please do not be tempted to use a nonfat sour cream. The reduced-fat version is made naturally with milk as well as cream for less fat content; the nonfat is loaded with stabilizers and preservatives.

2 tablespoons reduced-fat sour cream

2 teaspoons mayonnaise

$1/3$ cup low-fat buttermilk

$3/4$ teaspoon freshly squeezed lemon juice

1 tablespoon minced fresh dill

1 tablespoon minced fresh chives

2 teaspoons finely chopped fresh parsley

$1/2$ clove garlic, crushed through a press

Salt and freshly ground black pepper

In a small bowl, whisk together the sour cream and mayonnaise until thoroughly blended. Whisk in the buttermilk and lemon juice until incorporated.

Stir in the dill, chives, parsley, and garlic. Season with salt and pepper to taste.

# Tarragon Chicken Salad with Dried Cherries, Walnuts, and Grapes

## Serves 2

Elegant and enticing, this lovely chicken salad is lightened with yogurt standing in for most of the mayonnaise without sacrificing any flavor. As is true of any salad, the quality of the oil and vinegar will make it or break it. If you can find Banyuls vinegar from the south of France, it offers a mellow fruity flavor; otherwise, sherry vinegar, which is similar though a litte less subtle, is a good choice here. Feel free to dress up the plate with any other favorite vegetables you have on hand.

5 to 6 ounces cooked chicken, such as leftover from a rotisserie chicken

1/4 cup plain yogurt, preferably low-fat Greek-style or goat's milk

1 tablespoon mayonnaise

1 teaspoon Dijon mustard

2 teaspoons minced fresh tarragon, 1 teaspoon dried tarragon, or 1 tablespoon minced fresh dill

Salt and freshly ground black pepper

1/4 cup dried cherries, halved if large, and/or currants

3 tablespoons chopped walnuts, toasted (see note)

16 seedless red grapes, halved

4 cups mixed baby lettuces and/or arugula

1 tablespoon Banyuls or sherry wine vinegar

2 tablespoons extra virgin olive oil

Remove any skin from the chicken. Cut off any bits of fat or gristle. Cut the meat into 1/2-inch dice.

In a medium bowl, whisk together the yogurt, mayonnaise, mustard, and tarragon. Season with salt and pepper to taste. Add the chicken and toss to coat. Add the dried cherries, walnuts, and grapes. Fold gently to mix.

In a large bowl, toss the greens with the vinegar and oil to coat lightly. Divide between 2 plates and scoop the chicken salad on top.

NOTE: To toast the nuts, preheat the oven to 325°F. Place the nuts in a single layer in a small baking dish and toast for 5 to 7 minutes, until fragrant and very lightly browned.

# Gingered Beet and Scallop Salad

Serves 4

Ginger, which is a natural digestive aid, pairs beautifully with the mild sweetness of both the scallops and the beets. Use either red beets or golden beets, or, for a gorgeous presentation, half of each. Just be sure to keep them separate when you toss them with the vinegar, because the red ones will bleed. This delightful salad makes a perfect starter for a very special dinner.

4 small or 3 medium beets

6 large diver's scallops (8 to 10 ounces)

1/3 cup extra virgin olive oil

1 tablespoon finely minced fresh ginger

1 shallot, minced

1 1/2 teaspoons toasted walnut oil

1 tablespoon sherry wine vinegar

1 teaspoon freshly squeezed lemon juice

Salt and freshly ground black pepper

4 ounces mixed spring greens (mesclun) or arugula (about 4 cups)

Preheat the oven to 400°F. Wrap the beets in aluminum foil and roast for about 45 minutes, until tender. Let stand, wrapped, until cool enough to handle. The skins should slip right off. Cut the beets into about 1/2-inch dice.

Remove the little muscle from the side of the scallops and cut each horizontally into 2 or 3 slices about 1/4 inch thick. Pat dry. In a nonstick skillet, heat 1 tablespoon of the olive oil. Add the scallops and sauté over medium-high heat for about 2 minutes, until lightly browned. Turn over and sauté for 1 to 2 minutes on the second side. Remove to a plate.

Pour the remaining olive oil into the skillet and set over low heat. Add the ginger and shallot and cook for 30 to 60 seconds, just until fragrant. Scrape into a bowl and whisk in the walnut oil, vinegar, and lemon juice. Season with salt and pepper to taste.

Arrange a small bouquet of the greens to one side of each of 4 salad plates. Arrange the scallops in the center of the plate, with a little pile of roasted beets at the side. Drizzle a little of the vinaigrette over the scallops and greens, and serve.

# Tuscan Tuna and Bean Salad

## Serves 4 to 6

The Tuscans have their own beans—often those big fat white beans called cannellini—but here in the United States, I love experimenting with the wonderful variety of heirloom beans sold at Rancho Gordo (www.ranchogordo.com). Of course, you can open a can for convenience, and there is nothing wrong with that. But if digestibility is an issue, try cooking your own (see page 162) with these fresh crop beauties, and you'll see the difference in an instant.

1/4 cup extra virgin olive oil

1 tablespoon sherry wine vinegar

1 1/2 teaspoons freshly squeezed lemon juice

Salt and freshly ground black pepper

2 tablespoons finely chopped red onion or
  minced shallot

1/2 red bell pepper, peeled and diced

1 clove garlic, crushed through a press

2 tablespoons chopped fresh parsley

3 1/2 cups home-cooked or canned beans, preferably
  organic, rinsed and drained (see note)

1 (5-ounce) can light tuna packed in olive oil,
  drained

In a large bowl, whisk together the olive oil, vinegar, and lemon juice. Season with salt and pepper to taste. Add the red onion, bell pepper, garlic, and 1 1/2 tablespoons of the parsley.

Add the beans and toss to mix. Crumble the tuna over the beans and fold to mix. Sprinkle the remaining 1/2 tablespoon parsley on top. Serve slightly chilled or at room temperature.

NOTE: If using canned beans, use 2 (15-ounce) cans. Opt for cannellini beans or a mix of cannellini and black beans. If cooking your own (see Best Pot of Beans, page 162), try Rancho Gordo's speckled palomino beans; they're sure to stimulate conversation. Avoid red kidney beans; these contain a chemical that can cause stomachaches and inhibits the absorption of the vital nutrient folate.

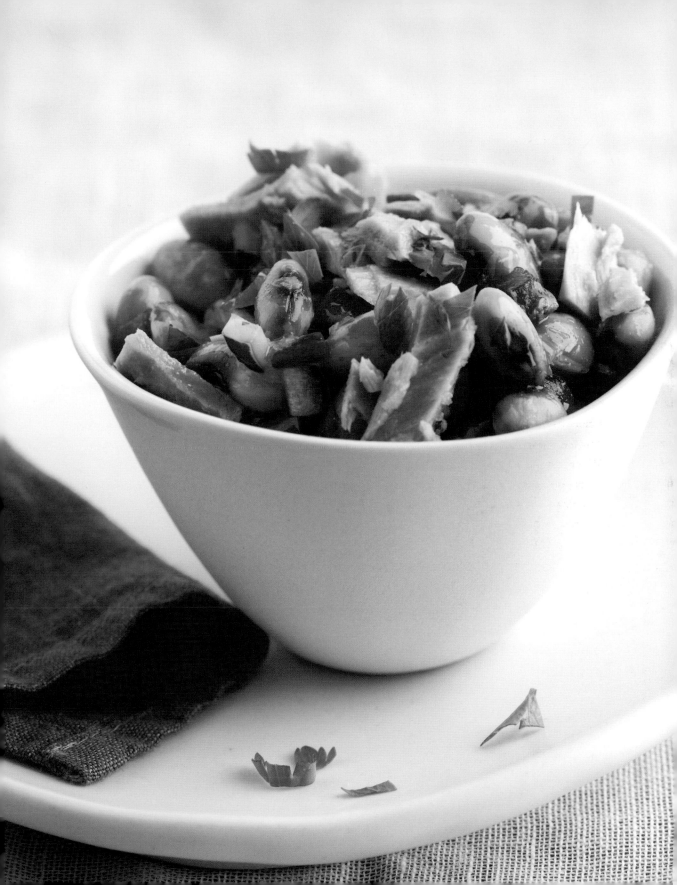

# Santa Fe Salmon Salad with Green Fairy Dressing

Serves 4

We often think of salads as mixed up, tossed mélanges, but colorful composed salads, with separate but synergistic elements coming together on a beautiful and tantalizing plate, are my favorites. Serve this Southwestern-inspired salad with baked corn tortillas, one per person. And if you tolerate fresh tomatoes, by all means, add a few wedges to each plate.

1 1/2 pounds center-cut salmon fillet, skinned and divided into 4 equal pieces (about 5 ounces each)

Salt and freshly ground black pepper

2 teaspoons freshly squeezed lemon juice

3 tablespoons extra virgin olive oil

4 corn tortillas

3/4 teaspoon ground cumin

Black Bean and Corn Salsa with Cilantro and Lime (page 66)

Green Fairy Dressing (recipe follows)

1 small Persian cucumber, peeled and sliced paper thin

1 (10-ounce) package baby spinach

Season the salmon with salt and pepper. Drizzle 1 teaspoon of the lemon juice and 1 1/2 teaspoons of the olive oil over the fish. Steam on an oiled rack over boiling water for 8 to 10 minutes, until just cooked through but still moist. Or grill for 5 to 6 minutes per side, if you prefer. (The salmon can be cooked up to a day in advance.)

Preheat the oven to 375°F. Cut each tortilla into 4 wedges and arrange in a single layer on a baking sheet. Coat lightly with cooking spray. Dust with the cumin and 3/4 teaspoon salt. Toast without turning for about 10 minutes, until crisp but not brown.

Meanwhile, prepare the salsa and dressing and set aside.

In a large bowl, toss the cucumber with the remaining 1 teaspoon lemon juice and remaining 1 1/2 teaspoons olive oil. Season generously with salt and pepper. Add the spinach and toss to coat lightly.

Divide the spinach and cucumbers among 4 large plates. Set the salmon on top of the salad and garnish each piece with a dollop of the dressing. Add about 1/2 cup of the salsa to each plate. Decorate the plates with the baked tortilla chips. Pass the remaining dressing on the side.

## GREEN FAIRY DRESSING

Makes about 1¹/₄ cups

While this pale green dressing was inspired by
the classic Green Goddess, it's much simpler
and gossamer light. It is a lovely topping for fish,
shrimp, or even spinach salad, and I've also found
it to be a superb and very popular dip with fresh
vegetables or chips.

1 small avocado
¹/₂ cup plain, low-fat yogurt
¹/₃ cup fresh Thai basil leaves
2 teaspoons freshly squeezed lemon juice
1¹/₂ teaspoons minced shallot
Salt and freshly ground black pepper

Scoop the avocado from its skin into a food processor or blender. Add the yogurt, basil, lemon
juice, and shallot. Whirl until light and very
smooth. Season with salt and pepper to taste.

# SEAFOOD

# Baked Flounder over Fennel Niçoise

Serves 4

Flounder is a tender, mild white fish that usually pleases everyone and takes well to many different flavorings and sauces. Here, it is cooked simply on a bed of fennel seasoned with flavors typical to the south of France and topped with a dusting of crisp bread crumbs to enhance the texture. Serve right from the baking dish or plate and bring to the table. Accompany the dish with lightly buttered orzo or rice, allowing $1/2$ cup per person.

3 cups diced fresh fennel ($1^1/2$ large bulbs)

1 small leek, white and tender green parts, thinly sliced

3 tablespoons extra virgin olive oil

$1/3$ cup coarsely chopped pitted kalamata olives

$1^1/2$ teaspoons grated orange zest

$1/3$ cup dry vermouth mixed with $1/2$ cup water

$1/4$ cup freshly squeezed orange juice

4 skinned flounder fillets (about 4 ounces each)

Salt and freshly ground black pepper

$1/3$ cup panko bread crumbs

Preheat the oven to 375°F.

In a flameproof gratin dish or large skillet, sauté the fennel and leek in $2^1/2$ tablespoons of the olive oil over medium-high heat for about 5 minutes, until softened. Reduce the heat to medium.

Add the olives, orange zest, vermouth and water, and orange juice. Reduce to a simmer, cover, and cook for 3 to 5 minutes, until the fennel is soft.

Arrange the fish fillets on top of the fennel. Season lightly with salt and pepper. Sprinkle the panko crumbs over the flounder and drizzle the remaining $1^1/2$ teaspoons olive oil over the crumbs.

Bake for 15 to 18 minutes, until the fish is just cooked through and the crumbs are lightly colored. Run under the broiler for the last minute or two for a browner top.

# Cod Tenderloins with Ragout of
# Shiitakes and Pea Shoots

Serves 4

Cod is an extremely lean, meaty fish that is inherently mild. Here the fish is coated with seasoned yogurt to keep it moist and crispy panko bread crumbs for added texture. I derived the idea for the easy mushroom and pea shoot adornment from a Thomas Keller recipe in his wonderful cookbook *Ad Hoc at Home*.

4 cod "tenderloins" (see note), about
    4$^1$/$_2$ ounces each

Salt and freshly ground black pepper

$^1$/$_3$ cup plain yogurt

1$^1$/$_2$ teaspoons Dijon mustard

$^1$/$_2$ teaspoon fresh thyme leaves

1 clove garlic, crushed through a press

$^3$/$_4$ cup panko bread crumbs

2 tablespoons extra virgin olive oil

Ragout of Shiitakes and Pea Shoots (recipe
    follows), for garnish

Lemon wedges, for garnish (optional)

Preheat the oven to 400°F. Season the cod with salt and pepper.

In a small bowl, whisk together the yogurt, mustard, thyme, and garlic. Brush all over the fish. Let stand for 10 to 15 minutes. Roll the tenderloins in the panko bread crumbs to coat.

In a large cast iron or other ovenproof skillet, warm the oil over medium heat. Add the tenderloins and cook for 3 to 4 minutes, until the crumbs are golden brown. Carefully turn the fish over.

Transfer the skillet to the oven and roast for 6 to 7 minutes, until the cod is just done. For nicer browning, run the top under the broiler for 30 to 60 seconds at the end.

Meanwhile, prepare the ragout. Spoon the shiitakes and pea shoots on top of the fish, along with a little bit of broth. Garnish with lemon wedges for anyone who can tolerate an extra spritz of lemon juice.

NOTE: Some markets sell what is labeled "cod tenderloins." These are thick strips of cod fillet about 1$^1$/$_2$ inches thick, 2 inches wide, and 4 to 5 inches long, much like a pork tenderloin. If you don't see them in your market, ask your fishmonger to cut some for you, or trim them yourself. If you have to buy extra fish to get the tenderloins, save the remainder for soup or chowder.

## RAGOUT OF SHIITAKES AND PEA SHOOTS

Serves 4

This marvelous vegetable garnish cooks in just minutes. While it is especially nice with fish, it could easily dress up a tender chicken cutlet, as well.

6 ounces fresh shiitake mushrooms

1 small shallot, minced

1 1/2 tablespoons unsalted butter or extra virgin olive oil

1/4 cup reduced-sodium chicken broth

4 ounces young pea shoots, preferably organic

Salt and freshly ground black pepper

Remove the stems from the shiitakes and discard. Thinly slice the caps.

In a wide or deep skillet, cook the sliced shiitakes and shallot in the butter over medium heat for about 2 minutes, until the shallot is soft and fragrant.

Pour in the chicken broth and heat for a few seconds. Remove from the heat. Add the pea shoots and toss to mix well; they should wilt only slightly. Season with salt and pepper.

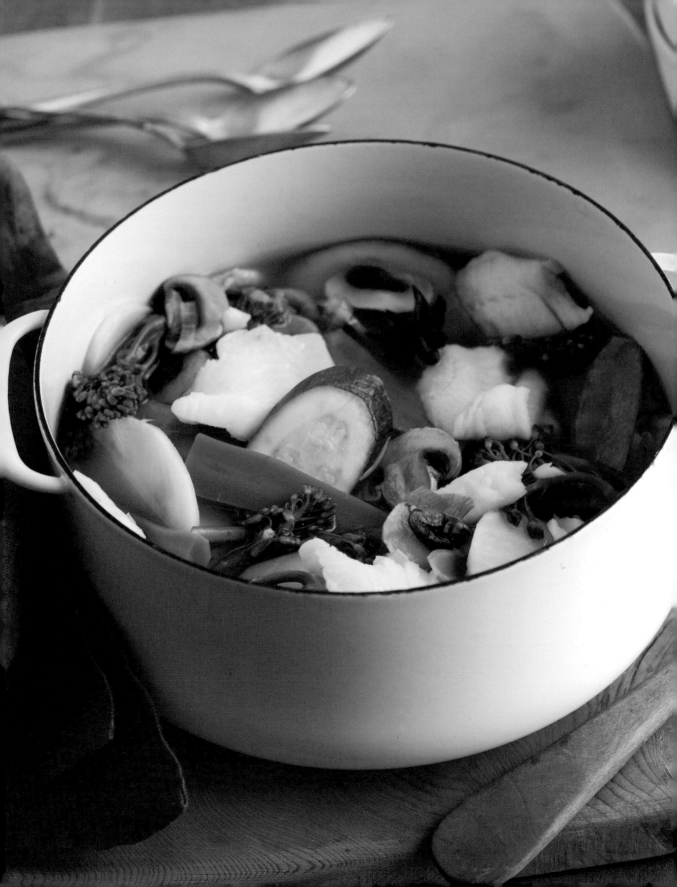

# Barigoule of Spring Vegetables with Fillet of Flounder

Serves 2

Light and aromatic, this lovely one-dish meal in a bowl is a cross between a soup and a stew. It won't weigh you down, and cooking time is little more than 10 minutes. While the small vegetables called for here are easiest to find in spring, it's a dish you really can make year-round simply by shopping carefully. Because it's so simple, using homemade stock will really make a difference.

2 cups Easy Rotisserie Chicken Stock (page 87), or any reduced-sodium chicken broth, diluted with 1 cup water

3 slices fresh ginger

3 wide strips lemon zest

$1^1/_2$ star anise pods

1 medium-small leek, white and tender green parts, thinly sliced

1 small turnip, peeled and thinly sliced

1 medium-small Yukon gold potato, peeled and thinly sliced

1 medium carrot, peeled, halved crosswise, and thinly sliced lengthwise

8 thin Broccolini or baby broccoli florets, trimmed to about 2 inches long

1 small zucchini, cut crosswise diagonally into 8 oval pieces

3 white button mushrooms or shiitake caps, thinly sliced

16 snow pea pods, ends trimmed

8 ounces skinned flounder fillets, cut into 2-inch squares or rectangles

In a large stainless steel skillet or enameled paella pan, combine the diluted chicken stock with the ginger, lemon zest, and star anise. Bring to a bare simmer and let steep over very low heat for 10 minutes.

Add the leek, turnip, potato, and carrot. Simmer, partially covered, over medium-low heat for 5 minutes. Add the Broccolini florets, zucchini, and mushrooms. Simmer, partially covered, for 3 minutes longer.

Add the pea pods and flounder, cover, and cook for 2 to 3 minutes, until the flounder is just cooked through. To serve, divide the fish and vegetables between 2 soup plates. Ladle the hot broth over all.

# Grilled Halibut with Black Bean and Corn Salsa

Serves 4

Fish is always a good choice for lightness and digestibility, and halibut is particularly good for picky seafood eaters because it has a mild, clean flavor. For an attractive presentation, be sure to rotate the fish on the grill to produce crosshatched marks, and spoon the bright-colored bean and corn salsa on top. You may also allow yourself $1/2$ cup of steamed rice and a crisp green salad with a wedge of avocado.

$1 1/2$ pounds halibut steaks, $3/4$ to 1 inch thick

$1/2$ teaspoon salt

$1/4$ teaspoon smoked paprika, preferably pimentón de la Vera

$1/8$ teaspoon freshly ground black pepper

1 tablespoon extra virgin olive oil

Black Bean and Corn Salsa with Cilantro and Lime (page 66)

Lime wedges, for garnish

Divide the steaks into 4 equal portions. Season on both sides with the salt, paprika, and pepper. Brush the olive oil over the fish.

Grill over a medium-hot fire on a barbecue grill or broil about 4 inches from the heat for 5 to 6 minutes, rotating 90 degrees halfway through to create those nice crosshatch marks. Turn over and repeat on the second side, cooking for 10 to 12 minutes total, until the fish is just opaque in the center but still juicy.

Remove the steaks from the heat and let stand for a couple of minutes. Prepare the salsa.

Serve each piece of fish with $1/2$ cup of the salsa. Garnish with a wedge of lime.

# Pistachio-Crusted Salmon with Braised Cabbage

### Serves 4

Choose wild Alaskan salmon, if you can, for this dish; it's leaner than farm raised and has a deep, rich flavor. What's particularly nice about this recipe is that you prepare it well ahead so the fish can marinate and then just pop it into the oven at the last minute, which makes a perfect plan for entertaining.

1¼ pounds center-cut salmon fillets, 1 inch thick, skin removed

2 teaspoons ground coriander seed

½ teaspoon demerara or turbinado sugar

Sea salt and freshly ground black pepper

2 tablespoons Dijon mustard

2½ tablespoons plus 2 teaspoons sunflower oil

1 tablespoon plus 2 teaspoons freshly squeezed lemon juice

1 large shallot, thinly sliced

6 cups shredded cabbage (about ¾ pound)

2 teaspoons rice vinegar or cider vinegar

¼ cup shelled and roasted pistachio nuts, coarsely ground

Set the salmon skinned side down in a small glass baking dish or pie pan. Season with 1 teaspoon of the ground coriander, the sugar, and ¼ teaspoon each salt and pepper. In a small bowl, whisk together the mustard with 2 teaspoons each of the sunflower oil and lemon juice. Spoon over the fish and spread over the top. Cover the fish with plastic wrap or aluminum foil, making sure it doesn't touch the mustard coating. Refrigerate for at least 1 hour and preferably up to 8 hours.

Up to 3 hours in advance, swirl the remaining 2½ tablespoons oil in a 10-inch cast iron skillet or other ovenproof pan and set it over medium heat. Add the shallot and cook for 30 seconds. Add the cabbage and toss to coat with the oil. Season with the remaining 1 teaspoon coriander, 1 teaspoon salt, and ¼ teaspoon pepper. Cook, tossing, for 5 to 7 minutes, until wilted and starting to turn golden. Add the vinegar and ¼ cup water. Continue to cook, stirring, for 5 to 7 minutes longer, until the cabbage is almost tender and most of the liquid has evaporated. Remove from the heat.

When you're ready to cook the salmon, preheat the oven to 375°F. Stir the remaining 1 tablespoon lemon juice and 2 tablespoons water into the cabbage and make a shallow bed in the center; set the salmon on top. Sprinkle the ground pistachios over the salmon to coat. Roast, uncovered, for 12 to 15 minutes, until the fish is just barely opaque in the center. Let stand for 2 to 3 minutes to finish cooking before serving.

# Grilled Spanish Mackerel with Gingered Mango Salsa

Serves 4

Nothing could be lighter, more refreshing, or more colorful than this easy warm-weather dish. Serve with $1/2$ cup—no more—steamed brown rice and as much grilled asparagus as you wish.

$1^1/4$ pounds Spanish mackerel or California sea
    bass fillets
Sea salt and freshly ground black pepper
1 teaspoon freshly squeezed lemon juice
2 teaspoons chopped fresh ginger
About 2 teaspoons extra virgin olive oil
Gingered Mango Salsa (recipe follows)

Season the fish lightly with sea salt and pepper. Sprinkle on the lemon juice and scatter the ginger over the top. Drizzle lightly with olive oil. Cover with plastic wrap and set aside at room temperature for 20 to 30 minutes, or refrigerate for a couple of hours.

Shortly before you're ready to serve, prepare the salsa. Then get the grill ready, oiling the rack before lighting the fire. You can also grill the fish on an oiled stovetop grill pan. Set the fish meaty side down and grill over medium-high heat for 3 minutes. Turn over carefully; most of the ginger will fall off, which is fine. Grill skin side down for 4 to 5 minutes, until the fish is just cooked through but still juicy.

Divide the fish into 4 portions. Lift the meat off the skin, if it hasn't come off already, and spoon $1/2$ cup of the salsa over each serving.

## GINGERED MANGO SALSA

Makes 2 cups

One way to avoid acid reflux is to eat easily digestible foods. While green bell peppers are typically "repeaters," red bell peppers, which are simply ripe versions of the green, are much friendlier. Removing the peel makes them even lighter and easier to digest. You can make this lovely salsa a couple of hours in advance, but for best flavor, chop the cilantro and add at the last moment. Its volatile oils disappear quickly.

$1/4$ large red bell pepper
$1^1/2$ cups finely diced ripe mango ($1^1/2$ to
    2 mangoes, depending on size)
1 teaspoon finely grated fresh ginger
$1/8$ teaspoon salt
2 teaspoons extra virgin olive oil
$1/4$ cup coarsely chopped fresh cilantro

Using a swivel-bladed vegetable peeler, remove the outer skin from the bell pepper; it will come off very easily. Cut the pepper into fine ($1/4$-inch) dice; there should be about $1/2$ cup.

In a small bowl, toss the bell pepper with the mango, ginger, salt, and olive oil. Shortly before serving, stir the cilantro into the salsa.

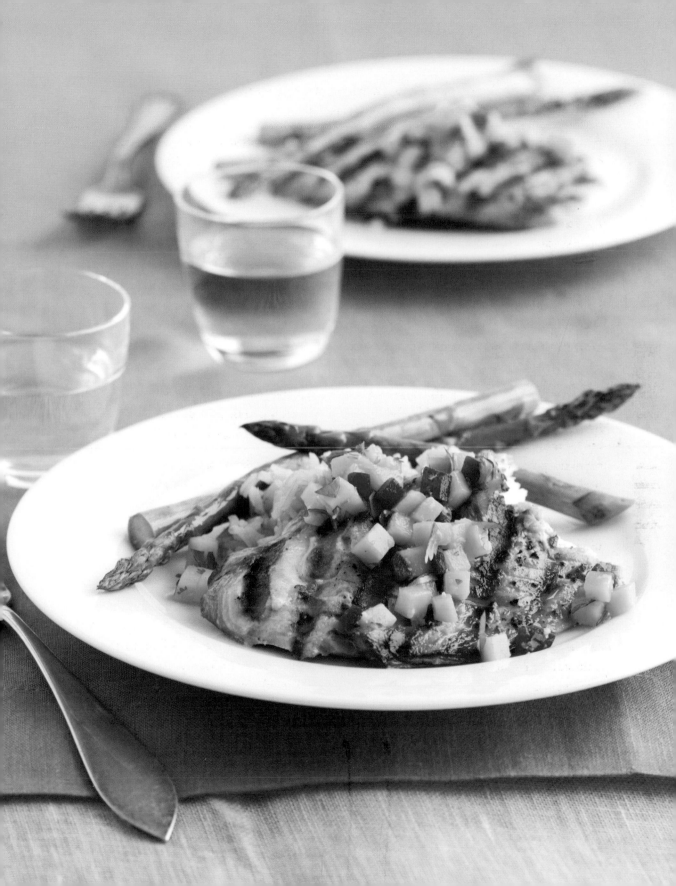

# Salmon Filet Mignon with Herb Butter

Serves 4

The only work involved in this lovely dish is "assembling" the salmon steaks, so read the first step, and if it doesn't sound like your kind of activity, ask your fishmonger to do it for you. Most of the butter seeps out after basting the fish with the flavorful herbs. Serve the fish as is, with a drizzle of the melted butter on the bottom of the dish, or set on top of a dollop of Romesco Sauce (page 74). Accompany with $1/2$ cup brown rice or a few small new potatoes and steamed lacinato kale or asparagus. Garnish with a lemon wedge.

2 (8-ounce) salmon steaks, 1 inch thick

1 tablespoon freshly squeezed lemon juice

$1/2$ teaspoon salt

$1/8$ teaspoon freshly ground black pepper

3 tablespoons unsalted butter, at room temperature

3 tablespoons finely chopped fresh chervil
    or parsley

$1 1/2$ tablespoons minced fresh chives

Olive oil

Divide the salmon steaks in half lengthwise, cutting on each side of the center bone to remove the fillets from each steak. Use your fingertips or tweezers to pull out any remaining pin bones. Cut into the center of the thicker part to within ¾ inch of the end without cutting all the way through so that the fillet can be opened up into one long strip. Repeat with the other 3 fillets.

Place the 4 salmon strips skin side down on a baking sheet. Drizzle the lemon juice over the fish and season with the salt and pepper.

In a small bowl, combine the butter, chervil, and chives. If the herb butter is very soft, refrigerate for a few minutes until it sets up but is still malleable. Spread over the salmon, leaving about a 1 inch-margin at the thinner end. Roll up loosely like pinwheels and secure with a couple of wooden toothpicks. You will have 4 rolls. (The dish can be prepared to this point up to 8 hours in advance, wrapped well, and stored in the refrigerator. Even if you are baking immediately, refrigerate for at least 10 minutes to firm up the filling.)

Preheat the oven to 375°F. Arrange the salmon tenderloins in a small oiled baking dish. Brush them lightly with olive oil and season with additional salt and pepper. Cover with aluminum foil and bake for 15 minutes. Uncover, turn over carefully, and bake for 5 to 8 minutes, until the salmon is just opaque in the center but still moist. Remove the toothpicks and peel off the skin, if you like, before serving.

# Shrimp-Stuffed Tilapia

Serves 4

Succulent and tasty, an Asian-inspired shrimp topping turns ordinary tilapia into a very nice fish, indeed. Thinly sliced pickled ginger, the kind used for sushi, comprises the secret ingredient here. The fish and shrimp together offer a substantial amount of protein, so all you'll need as an accompaniment are a couple of nice vegetables. Steamed or grilled asparagus and summer squash would be good choices.

2 tilapia fillets (8 to 10 ounces each)

Salt and freshly ground black pepper

$1/3$ cup pickled sushi ginger ($1 3/4$ to 2 ounces)

2 tablespoons sliced scallion, white part only

1 meaty strip of nitrate-free bacon, diced

$1/2$ pound shrimp, shelled, deveined, and tails removed

3 ounces sliced water chestnuts (about $1/2$ cup)

2 tablespoons minced chives

1 small shallot, minced

$1/3$ cup dry vermouth or white wine

1 tablespoon freshly squeezed lemon juice

1 tablespoon unsalted butter

Preheat the oven to 375°F. Pat the tilapia fillets dry. Cut them lengthwise down the center to make 4 long fillets. Season lightly with salt and pepper.

In a food processor, combine the ginger, scallion, and bacon. Pulse to chop. Add the shrimp and $1/4$ teaspoon salt. Pulse about 8 times to chop the shrimp. Add the water chestnuts and pulse another 8 to 10 times to chop the water chestnuts. Add the chives and whirl for a few seconds to blend. Spread the shrimp paste over the top of the tilapia fillets.

Butter a flameproof gratin dish or oven-proof skillet. Sprinkle the shallot over the bottom of the dish and arrange the fish on top. Pour the vermouth, lemon juice, and 2 tablespoons water into the dish. Bring to a simmer on top of the stove. Cover loosely with a sheet of buttered waxed paper.

Transfer to the oven and bake for 10 minutes. Remove the paper and bake for 6 to 8 minutes longer, until the fish is just cooked through. Run the dish under a broiler for 2 to 3 minutes, until glazed and lightly browned.

With a slotted spatula, transfer the fish to a platter or plates. Strain the juices left in the dish into a small skillet. Boil until reduced to 4 or 5 tablespoons. Remove from the heat and whisk in the tablespoon of butter. Spoon the juices over the fish and serve.

# Coconut Shrimp with Watermelon and Yellow Tomato Salad

## Serves 4

While they are decidedly a treat, because these sweet, succulent shrimp are baked rather than fried, they can be part of the Acid Reflux Solution, especially since the fat in coconut is so easy to digest. For the most impressive presentation, choose the largest shrimp you can find; if you have access to colossal (12 to 16 per pound), increase the cooking time to 12 to 15 minutes. Serve with Watermelon and Yellow Tomato Salad.

20 jumbo or 16 colossal shrimp, peeled and
   deveined, tails intact
3 egg whites
2 tablespoons Dijon mustard
2 tablespoons sunflower oil
1/2 cup cornstarch
1 1/2 cups sweetened flaked coconut
Watermelon and Yellow Tomato Salad
   (recipe follows)

Preheat the oven to 425°F.

Rinse the shrimp and pat dry. Slit down the back without cutting all the way through, leaving the tails intact, to butterfly the shrimp. Press open gently.

In a wide bowl, whisk together the egg whites and mustard until thoroughly blended. Slowly whisk in the oil. Pile the cornstarch on a sheet of waxed paper. Put the coconut on another sheet. Dip the shrimp in the mustard mixture, then dredge in the cornstarch and shake off any excess. Dip in the mustard again and roll in the coconut to coat completely, pressing gently to help the shreds adhere. Arrange the coated shrimp on a lightly greased sturdy baking sheet.

Bake for 5 minutes. Carefully turn the shrimp over and bake for 4 to 5 minutes on the second side, until the coconut is lightly browned and the shrimp are opaque throughout.

While the shrimp are baking, prepare the salad.

Serve the hot shrimp with the room-temperature watermelon and tomato salad.

*Continued*

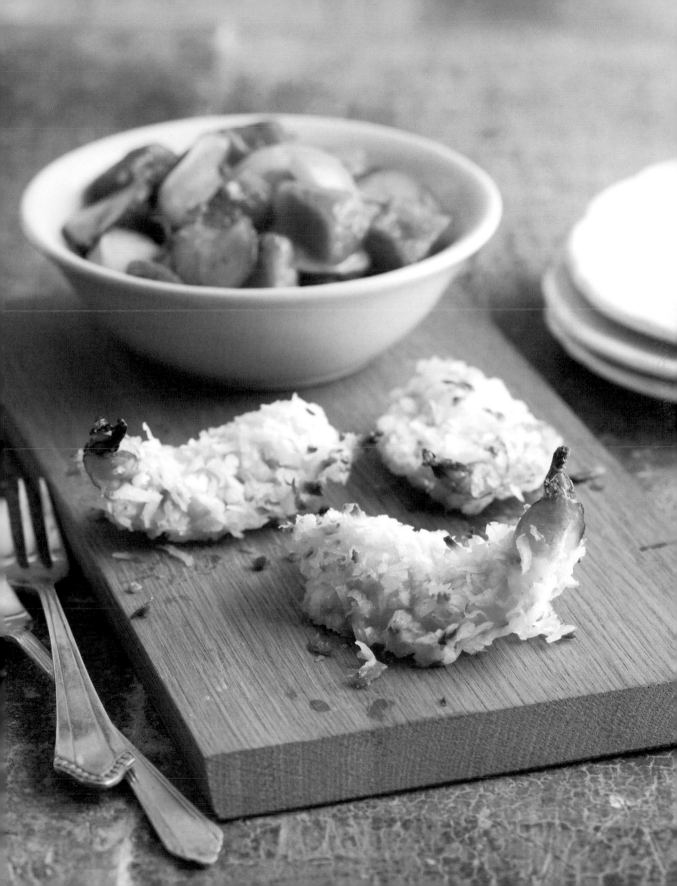

## WATERMELON AND YELLOW TOMATO SALAD
Serves 4

Though there is no scientific evidence to explain it, some people who suffer from acid reflux have a lot of trouble with the acid in tomatoes. However, yellow tomatoes are distinctly lower in acid than the red ones, and there are cultivars, which you might want to grow, that are essentially acid free. This recipe is loaded with fiber and both lycopene and beta-carotene, a pair of powerful antioxidants.

2 pounds seedless watermelon

1 pound yellow tomatoes

1 small seedless or 1 medium pickling cucumber, very thinly sliced (about 1 cup)

1 1/2 teaspoons demerara or turbinado sugar

1/2 teaspoon salt

1 1/2 tablespoons balsamic vinegar

1 1/2 tablespoons extra virgin olive oil

1 1/2 tablespoons slivered fresh basil

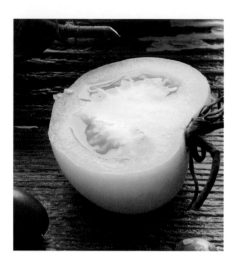

Remove the watermelon rind and cut the flesh into 1-inch chunks; there will be about 4 cups. Core the tomatoes and cut into 3/4-inch dice; there will be about 2 cups.

In a pretty serving bowl, toss the watermelon, yellow tomatoes, and cucumber with the sugar, salt, balsamic vinegar, and olive oil. Let stand at room temperature for 10 to 15 minutes. Add the basil, toss, and serve. This salad gives off a lot of juice, so it's best to dish with a slotted spoon.

# POULTRY AND MEATS

# Asian Barbecued Chicken

## Serves 4

Traditionally used for pork barbecue, this no-fat-added technique works beautifully with chicken. The seasoned sauce imbues the meat with succulent flavor, while the pan of water underneath keeps it moist and tender. Serve with 1/2 cup steamed rice per person and baby bok choy or your favorite green leafy vegetable.

4 large or 8 small skinless, boneless chicken thighs
    (1 to 1 1/4 pounds total)

1/4 cup hoisin sauce

1 1/2 tablespoons soy sauce

1 1/2 tablespoons pale dry sherry

2 teaspoons honey

1 clove garlic, crushed through a press

1/4 teaspoon Chinese five-spice powder (see note)

Trim any fat or gristle off the chicken thighs. Open them up as flat as you can.

In a medium bowl, whisk together the hoisin sauce, soy sauce, sherry, honey, garlic, and five-spice powder. Add the chicken and marinate at room temperature, turning frequently, for up to 1 hour, or in the refrigerator for up to 3 hours.

Preheat the oven to 325°F. Arrange the chicken thighs on a rack set over a baking dish filled halfway with water. Brush with some of the marinade in the bowl and roast for 20 minutes. If the water in the pan is drying up, add some more. Brush the chicken again with the marinade, turn over, and brush the second side. Roast for 20 to 25 minutes longer, until the chicken is white throughout but still moist.

NOTE: Chinse five-spice powder is a marvelously aromatic blend of ground Sichuan peppercorns, star anise, fennel, cinnamon, and cloves. While in the past you had to make a trip to an Asian market to purchase the spice mixture, most of the major seasoning brands now carry the powder, so you can find it in your supermarket.

# Crispy Braised Chicken with Smoked Paprika

Serves 4 to 6

A naked chicken is not an attractive sight, but removing the skin along with all the fat that clings to it cuts your saturated fat calories by almost two-thirds. If you don't want to do it, ask your butcher; even at the supermarket, they will accommodate you. Next, the chicken is marinated to develop flavor; don't worry, the onions are tossed out at the end. And finally, it's dressed back up with a crispy coating of seasoned panko bread crumbs.

1 (3¼- to 3½-pound) chicken, preferably organic and free range, skinned

1½ teaspoons freshly squeezed lemon juice

1½ tablespoons extra virgin olive oil

Salt and freshly ground black pepper

1 teaspoon smoked paprika, preferably pimentón de la Vera

1 medium onion, sliced

6 to 8 fresh parsley sprigs

¼ cup dry vermouth

½ cup reduced-sodium chicken broth

½ cup panko bread crumbs

¼ teaspoon dried thyme

1 tablespoon unsalted butter

Press down firmly on the breastbone of the chicken with your palm to flatten it slightly. Set it splayed out, meaty side up, in a gratin dish or shallow flameproof baking dish. Rub all over with the lemon juice and olive oil. Season with 1 teaspoon salt, ¼ teaspoon pepper, and ½ teaspoon of the smoked paprika. Arrange the onion slices and parsley on top. Cover the pan snugly with plastic wrap and aluminum foil and let marinate at room temperature for 1 hour or in the refrigerator for up to 8 hours or even overnight. (If chilled, let stand at room temperature for 30 to 60 minutes before cooking.)

Preheat the oven to 375°F. Pour the vermouth and broth into the bottom of the dish around the chicken. Cover with foil. Bring to a simmer on top of the stove. Transfer to the oven and braise the chicken for 30 minutes. Remove from the oven; raise the temperature to 425°F.

In a small bowl, toss the panko crumbs with the thyme, remaining ½ teaspoon smoked paprika, ½ teaspoon salt, and ⅛ teaspoon pepper. Use tongs to remove and discard the onion and parsley. Sprinkle the seasoned crumbs over the chicken to coat the top and sides, pressing them gently to adhere. Return to the oven and roast uncovered for 15 to 20 minutes, until the chicken is just cooked through but still juicy and the crumbs are lightly colored.

Transfer the chicken to a platter. Strain the cooking juices into a small saucepan and boil until reduced to a scant ½ cup. Stir in the butter just until melted. Drizzle the sauce over the chicken or pass on the side.

# Spanish Chicken and Rice

### Serves 4

If my mother sees this recipe, I'm going to have a lot of explaining to do. It was a challenge to convey all the flavors of the traditional Cuban dish but keep the GERD components at bay. Lighter and leaner than the original, this dish can go from start to finish in roughly half an hour. The traditional rice used in this sort of Latin dish is a medium- or short-grain rice, like Spanish Bomba or an Italian risotto rice, such as Arborio. Any will deliver the chewy texture that makes this dish so pleasing. If asparagus is not in season, substitute 6 ounces marinated artichoke hearts, drained, quartered lengthwise, and blotted on paper towels to remove excess oil. Serve with a lovely green salad, such as Arugula and Hearts of Palm Salad (page 94).

12 ounces thick skinless, boneless chicken breasts

1 1/2 teaspoons ground cumin

1 1/2 teaspoons oregano

1 teaspoon smoked paprika, preferably pimentón de la Vera

Salt and freshly ground black pepper

1 yellow onion, chopped

3 tablespoons olive oil

1 clove garlic, chopped

1 cup short-grain rice, such as Bomba or Arborio

1 1/2 cups (about 14 ounces) diced peeled tomatoes, preferably Pomi brand (see note, page 132)

1/2 teaspoon saffron threads

3 cups Easy Rotisserie Chicken Stock (page 87), or any reduced-sodium chicken broth

2/3 cup frozen baby peas, thawed

1/2 cup Spanish pimiento-stuffed green olives

12 asparagus stalks, trimmed to about 6 inches

8 to 12 strips piquillo peppers or peeled, roasted red bell peppers, for garnish (see note, page 132)

Cut the chicken into 1-inch chunks. Toss in a bowl with 1/2 teaspoon each of the cumin, oregano, and smoked paprika. Season with salt and pepper. Set aside.

In a paella pan or large skillet, cook the onion in the olive oil over medium-high heat, stirring occasionally, for 3 to 5 minutes, until it just begins to color. Add the garlic and cook for 30 seconds, then add the chicken. Cook, stirring, for 2 to 3 minutes, until the chicken is mostly white outside.

Sprinkle on the rice and cook, stirring, for 2 to 3 minutes, until the rice is opaque. Add the tomatoes, the remaining 1 teaspoon each cumin and oregano, the remaining 1/2 teaspoon smoked paprika, the saffron, and 2 1/2 cups of the stock. Cover, reduce the heat to low, and cook for 15 minutes, stirring every 5 minutes. Season with salt and pepper to taste.

*Continued*

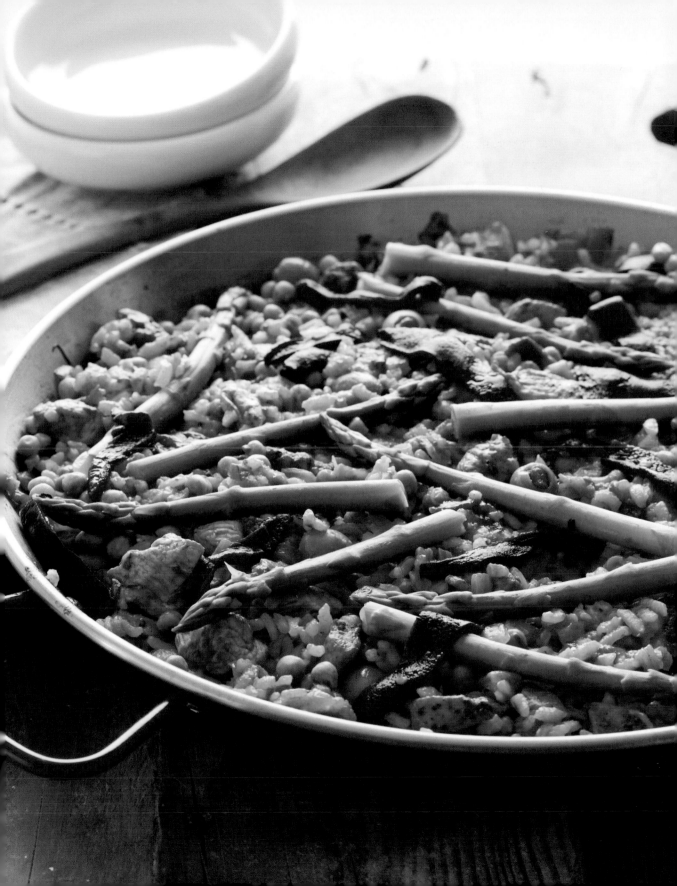

Stir in the remaining ½ cup stock, peas, and olives. Arrange the asparagus on top. Garnish with the strips of pepper. Cover, raise the heat to medium, and cook for 5 to 7 minutes, until the asparagus is just tender.

NOTE: When I can find it, I use Pomi brand cut-up tomatoes because the brand contains only one ingredient: tomatoes, with no added acid.

Piquillo peppers come in jars and offer a nice piquant but not hot note. Otherwise, ordinary peeled, roasted red bell peppers, which are available both jarred and in olive bars in many supermarkets, would do nicely.

# Chicken Cutlets with Arugula and Olive Sauce

### Serves 4 to 6

Because this pretty dish is served at room temperature, it's really perfect for casual entertaining. Yes, there are some tomatoes in this dish, but grape tomatoes are unusually sweet and low in acid; they should not cause a problem for most people. If you are particularly sensitive, even to fresh tomatoes, substitute diced yellow tomato, or simply omit them. Serve with a slice of whole-grain peasant bread to dip in the sauce.

1 1/2 pounds chicken cutlets or skinless, boneless chicken breasts, cut horizontally in half

Salt and freshly ground black pepper

2 teaspoons freshly squeezed lemon juice

4 1/2 tablespoons extra virgin olive oil

2 cups arugula, coarsely cut up

1 small shallot, minced

1 cup grape tomatoes, quartered (optional)

1/2 cup pitted kalamata olives, quartered

1 tablespoon balsamic vinegar

Lemon wedges, for garnish

Place the chicken cutlets between 2 sheets of waxed paper and pound lightly with a rolling pin to flatten evenly. Season both sides lightly with salt and pepper and sprinkle with 1 teaspoon of the lemon juice and 1 1/2 teaspoons of the olive oil. Let stand for 10 to 15 minutes.

Meanwhile, light a medium-hot fire in a barbecue grill or preheat a stovetop grill pan. Grill the chicken cutlets for 2 to 3 minutes per side, or until just cooked through. Transfer to a deep platter. Scatter the arugula over the warm chicken.

In a small saucepan, cook the shallot in the remaining 1/4 cup olive oil over medium heat for 30 seconds. Add the tomatoes and olives and stir to coat them with the oil. Stir in the balsamic vinegar and remaining 1 teaspoon lemon juice. Pour the warm sauce over the arugula and chicken. Garnish with lemon wedges, if you like. Serve warm or at room temperature.

# Rosemary-Fennel Chicken Cutlets

Serves 4

A blend of Mediterranean herbs turns simple chicken into a fresh-tasting dish that can be dressed up or down. For reflux sufferers, it may look as if there is a lot of garlic and oil in the recipe, but most comes off before cooking and just contributes lovely flavor. Serve with $^1/_2$ cup quinoa per person and steamed asparagus, baby broccoli, or zucchini.

4 chicken cutlets, 4 to 4$^1/_2$ ounces each

$^1/_4$ cup extra virgin olive oil

1 tablespoon freshly squeezed lemon juice

2 cloves garlic, crushed

2 teaspoons chopped fresh rosemary

1$^1/_2$ teaspoons fennel seed

$^1/_2$ teaspoon coarse salt

Freshly ground black pepper

Trim any fat or gristle from the chicken. If the cutlets are more than $^1/_2$ inch thick, pound them gently to flatten evenly. Place in a pie dish or deep platter.

In a mini food processor, combine the olive oil, lemon juice, garlic, rosemary, fennel seed, salt, and pepper to taste. Whirl for about 30 seconds to blend well. (If you don't have a small processor, whisk all the marinade ingredients together in a bowl.) Pour the marinade over the chicken and let stand at room temperature for about 30 minutes, or refrigerate for up to 3 hours.

Shortly before serving, light a medium-hot fire in a barbecue grill or preheat a stovetop grill pan. Scrape most of the marinade off the chicken. Grill, rotating to make crosshatched brown grill marks and turning once, for 3 to 4 minutes per side, until the chicken is just cooked through with no trace of pink in the center but is still juicy.

# Chicken Sukiyaki

Serves 4

Hot pots that are a sort of cross between a soup and a stew can be light and easy on the stomach. This one is very pretty and can be served in its deep skillet right at the table. No rice is served with sukiyaki; it contains its own noodles. I use Thai rice noodles or traditional Japanese cellophane noodles, made from a starchy vegetable. Both are gluten free and have a slippery texture.

Tatsoi, a spring green that has a pleasing, mild bite and can be eaten raw or cooked, is another Asian ingredient that can add extra flavor in place of the more usual spinach. To slice the chicken paper thin, place it in the freezer for 15 to 30 minutes, until it is almost frozen. Then use a sharp knife to slice it crosswise against the grain, cutting at a slight angle so the pieces are not too narrow.

6 ounces Thai rice noodles, or 4 ounces Japanese
    cellophane noodles (shirataki; see note,
      page 136)
3 cups Easy Rotisserie Chicken Stock (page 87),
    or any reduced-sodium chicken broth
1/3 cup mirin
1/4 cup soy sauce
1 tablespoon shredded fresh ginger
4 scallions, cut into 1 1/2-inch-long pieces
1 1/2 tablespoons peanut oil
1 large sweet onion, cut into rings about
    1/4 inch thick
6 ounces Chinese napa cabbage, cut crosswise into
    2-inch pieces
12 ounces skinless, boneless chicken breast, sliced
    paper thin
6 ounces fresh shiitake mushrooms, stemmed
4 ounces firm tofu, cut into about 1/2-inch slabs
5 to 6 ounces tatsoi or baby spinach, well rinsed

If using the Thai rice noodles, boil them in a medium saucepan of water for 5 minutes; drain and rinse. If using the cellophane noodles, soak them in a bowl of very hot water for 20 to 30 minutes, until softened.

In a large measuring cup or bowl, combine the stock, mirin, soy sauce, ginger, and scallions. Set aside.

Slick the bottom of a 16-inch deep skillet or large flameproof casserole with the oil. Arrange a single layer of the onion rings to cover the bottom of the pan (you may not need them all). Cook over medium-high heat, turning once, for 5 to 7 minutes, until they are softened and beginning to turn golden on one side. Reduce the heat to medium-low.

Pile the cabbage over the onions. Arrange a layer of chicken slices over the cabbage. Add the shiitake mushroom caps, a layer of the tofu, and finally the tatsoi. Pour the chicken

*Continued*

stock mixture over all, cover, and simmer for 5 minutes.

Add the noodles and simmer for 3 to 5 minutes longer, until the chicken is cooked through and all the vegetables are tender. To serve, divide the ingredients among 4 shallow soup bowls, then ladle on the stock.

NOTE: If the slippery texture of the Asian noodles doesn't appeal to you, you can substitute 4 ounces vermicelli, cooked in a saucepan of salted water for 4 to $4\frac{1}{2}$ minutes, until just barely tender.

# Turkey Shepherd's Pie

## Serves 4 to 6

No question, this would be even more delicious made traditionally with lamb or beef, but guess what? It wouldn't make you very happy a few hours later. You'll find that with the lightness of the turkey and the texture of all the vegetables, this goes down easy. Utilizing chunks of fresh turkey provides much better flavor and texture than ground.

1 yellow onion, diced

2 tablespoons extra virgin olive oil

3 tablespoons flour

2 cups turkey broth, Easy Rotisserie Chicken Stock (page 87), or any reduced-sodium chicken broth

1 teaspoon fresh thyme leaves, or

   $1/2$ teaspoon dried

$1/2$ teaspoon crushed dried sage

Sea salt and freshly ground black pepper

12 ounces white button or cremini mushrooms, quartered

1 cup diced carrots

$1/4$ pound green beans, cut into thirds

$11/4$ pounds thick-sliced turkey cutlets or skinless, boneless breast, cut into $3/4$-inch cubes

1 cup edamame (shelled soybeans), thawed if frozen

Buttermilk Mashed Potatoes with Parsnips (page 171)

Preheat the oven to 375°F.

In a large skillet or flameproof casserole, cook the onion in the olive oil over medium heat for about 5 minutes, until softened and golden. Sprinkle on the flour and cook, stirring, for 1 to 2 minutes, without allowing it to color. Whisk in the broth. Add the thyme and sage and bring to a boil, stirring until the liquid thickens. Reduce the heat to medium-low. Season generously with salt and pepper.

Add the mushrooms, carrots, and green beans. Simmer for 5 minutes. Add the turkey and edamame; simmer for 5 minutes longer. Transfer the turkey, vegetables, and sauce to a 9-inch round shallow casserole or deep pie dish. Mound the mashed potatoes and parsnips on top. Use the back of a large spoon to create decorative dips and swirls.

Bake the shepherd's pie for 25 minutes, or until the stew is bubbling and the edges of the potatoes are lightly browned on top.

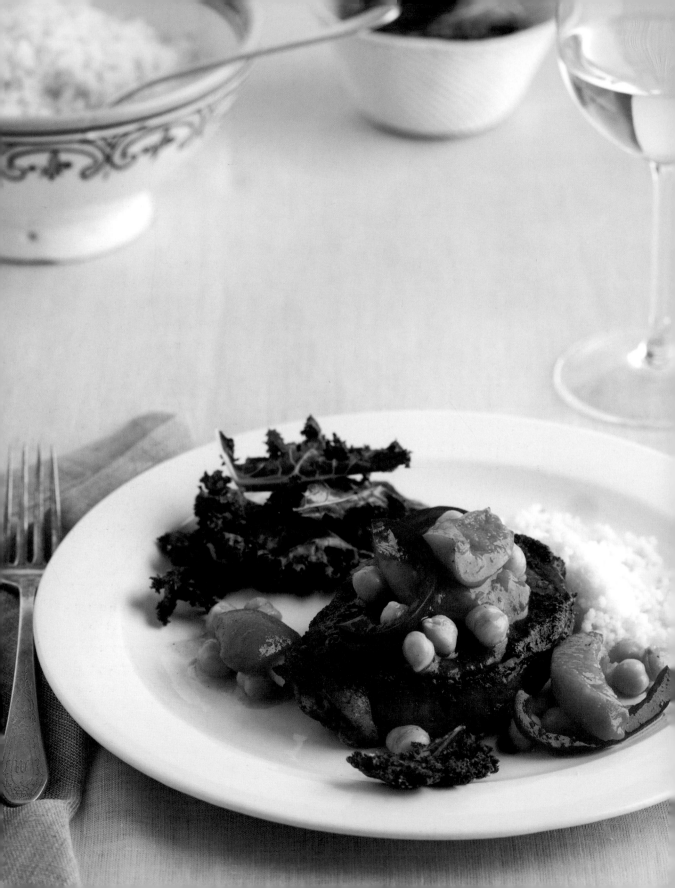

# Moroccan Spiced Pork Loin with Apricots and Chickpeas

### Serves 4

Pork is not a meat eaten in North Africa or the Middle East, but this dish celebrates the sweetly spiced seasonings of Morocco, which pair so beautifully with fruit and chickpeas. Choose a free-range, humanely raised brand, if you are able; the meat will have a healthier fat profile. Serve the chops with Frizzled Kale (page 173) and $1/2$ cup steamed couscous.

4 boneless pork loin chops, about 5 ounces each

1 teaspoon salt

1 teaspoon ground cumin

$1/2$ teaspoon cinnamon

$1/4$ teaspoon ground allspice

$1/8$ teaspoon freshly ground black pepper

1 clove garlic, crushed though a press

$1 1/2$ tablespoons extra virgin olive oil

1 cup vegetable or reduced-sodium chicken broth

1 (15- to 16-ounce) can chickpeas, preferably organic, rinsed and drained

$1/2$ red bell pepper, sliced (optional)

1 pound fresh apricots, peeled, quartered, and pitted, or 1 can apricot halves in light syrup, drained

$1 1/2$ tablespoons honey

1 teaspoon cornstarch

Parsley, for garnish

Trim any outer fat from the pork so it is as lean as possible. In a small bowl, combine the salt, cumin, cinnamon, allspice, pepper, and garlic. Stir in $1 1/2$ teaspoons of the olive oil to make a dry paste. Rub this over both sides of the pork chops and set aside at room temperature for 30 to 60 minutes.

Preheat the oven to 350°F. In a flameproof baking dish or ovenproof skillet, heat the remaining 1 tablespoon olive oil. Add the pork chops and brown over moderately high heat for $1 1/2$ to 2 minutes per side. Remove the meat to a plate.

Add $3/4$ cup of the stock to the dish and bring to a simmer, scraping up any browned bits from the bottom with a wooden spoon. Add the chickpeas, red pepper, and one-third of the apricots. Set the pork chops on top. Arrange the remaining apricots on top of the meat. Cover the dish and set in the oven.

Bake for about 25 minutes, or until the internal temperature of the chops registers 145° to 150°F. Remove the meat to a plate.

Stir the honey into the juices and bring to a boil. Blend the cornstarch with the remaining $1/4$ cup stock. Stir into the hot juices and boil, stirring, for 1 to 2 minutes, until the sauce thickens and clears. Spoon the chickpeas, red pepper, apricots, and sauce over the chops and serve garnished with parsley.

# Herb-Crusted Rack of Lamb with Savory White Beans

Serves 4 to 6

Rack of lamb used to be an enormous luxury, but excellent meat from Australia and New Zealand has made mild, sustainably raised lamb a good buy. Even better, if the rack is completely trimmed (frenched), as most are, you're getting a nugget of very lean meat and built-in portion control. What's especially nice about this recipe for entertaining is that you can prepare the lamb ahead of time and pop it in the oven just before dinner. Allow 3 small ribs per person and $1/2$ to $2/3$ cup beans. Also offer a steamed leafy green, such as chard or kale.

2 racks of lamb, about 1 pound each

$2^1/2$ tablespoons extra virgin olive oil

2 slices whole-grain bread

$1/4$ cup packed fresh parsley leaves

2 teaspoons fresh rosemary leaves or dried herbes de Provence

2 tablespoons Dijon mustard

Savory White Beans (recipe follows)

Make sure the racks are well trimmed of any external fat. With a sharp knife, lightly score the meaty side of the lamb in a diamond pattern; pat dry. Heat 1 tablespoon of the olive oil in a cast iron skillet just large enough to hold the racks, or use 2 pans if you need to. Add the lamb meaty side down and sauté over medium-high heat for 3 to 5 minutes, until lightly browned. Turn over and sauté for 1 to 2 minutes on the second side. Transfer to a small platter. Pour out any grease from the pan and wipe clean with paper towels. Let the meat cool for about 10 minutes.

Meanwhile, tear the bread into a small food processor. Add the parsley and rosemary. Pulse to chop coarsely, then process until the bread is ground to crumbs. Brush the mustard over the top and sides of the lamb. Pat the herbed crumbs over the lamb. Drizzle each rack lightly with the remaining $1^1/2$ tablespoons olive oil. The lamb can be roasted at this point or refrigerated for up to 8 hours; if chilled, let stand at room temperature for 1 hour before proceeding.

Preheat the oven to 400°F. Set the racks of lamb in the cast iron skillet or in a shallow baking pan and roast in the oven for 22 to 25 minutes, until the meat registers 135°F on a meat thermometer for medium-rare.

While the lamb is roasting, prepare the beans.

Let the lamb stand for a few minutes, then divide each rack into 3 large pieces of 3 ribs each, or carve to separate into chops. Serve with the beans.

## SAVORY WHITE BEANS

Serves 6

Beans are a very good food for people suffering from acid reflux because they are high in fiber and low in fat. That said, because they do produce gas, you want to enjoy them in moderation. You'll find the more often you eat them, the more digestible they become. Lamb and beans love each other, and this is a great shortcut recipe that doctors up the canned variety to excellent effect.

2 (14.5-ounce) cans cannellini beans, preferably
    organic, rinsed and drained

1 ounce diced lean pancetta

1 1/2 tablespoons extra virgin olive oil

1 cup finely diced carrot

1 cup finely diced fresh fennel or celery

1 1/2 teaspoons tomato paste

2 cups Easy Rotisserie Chicken Stock (page 87),
    or any reduced-sodium chicken broth

1 teaspoon winter savory or lemon thyme,
    or a mixture

1 small clove garlic, crushed through a press

Salt and freshly ground black pepper

Put the beans in a sieve and rinse under cold running water until the liquid runs clear. Drain well.

In a medium saucepan, cook the pancetta in the olive oil over medium heat for 3 to 5 minutes, until it begins to color lightly. Add the carrot and fennel, and cook for about 3 minutes longer, until slightly softened. Add the tomato paste and cook, stirring, for 1 to 2 minutes, until it darkens.

Pour in the stock and add the savory, garlic, and beans. Bring to a boil, crushing a few tablespoons of the beans with a wooden spatula or a fork. Reduce the heat, and simmer for 10 minutes, or until the liquid is reduced to a thick sauce. Season with salt and pepper to taste.

# Grass-Fed Beef and Portobello Blue Cheese Burgers

Serves 4

A burger is not what you'd expect to find in an acid reflux book. But my feeling is that the less food you have to give up, the easier it is to stick to the program. What you're really not supposed to eat is a lot of heavy saturated fat or high-glycemic foods, which is exactly what you get in a fast food burger and fries. And I'm sure you've felt the effects. I know I have.

This recipe uses grass-fed beef, which is leaner than ordinary meat and contains twice the amount of healthy omega-3s. After cooking, you're getting only about 3 ounces of meat. But with the grilled portobello on top and a surprise blue cheese filling, it's totally satisfying. Note the trick with trimming the roll to keep volume down. To complete the meal, top with Red and Green Ginger-Sesame Slaw (page 99) and serve with Baked Sweet Potato Fries (page 178).

1 pound lean, ground, grass-fed beef

Salt and freshly ground black pepper

2 ounces ($1/4$ cup) Roquefort cheese

2 tablespoons light whipped cream cheese

1 tablespoon minced fresh chives

4 portobello mushroom caps

1 tablespoon extra virgin olive oil

4 kaiser rolls

Season the beef lightly with salt and pepper. Divide into 4 equal portions. Then divide each portion in half and on a sheet of parchment or waxed paper, pat the beef into 8 very thin rounds about 4 inches in diameter.

In a small bowl, mash together the Roquefort, cream cheese, and chives until blended. Spread about 1 tablespoon of the cheese mixture over each of 4 rounds of beef, leaving at least a $1/4$-inch margin around the rim. Set the plain meat on top and pinch the edges to seal the cheese inside.

Season the mushrooms lightly with salt and pepper. Sprinkle the olive oil over the gills.

Cut out and discard a $1/2$-inch slice from the center of each bun. This will leave you with a trimmed down top and bottom.

Grill the mushrooms gill side down over a hot fire or on a grill pan on the stove for 3 minutes. Turn over and cook for 4 to 6 minutes longer, until they are softened and the juices begin to bubble up. Grill the burgers for about 3 minutes per side for medium-rare. Toast the buns for 1 to 2 minutes. To assemble, place each burger on a roll bottom. Add a mushroom cap, gill side down. Top with some slaw and set the tops of the rolls in place.

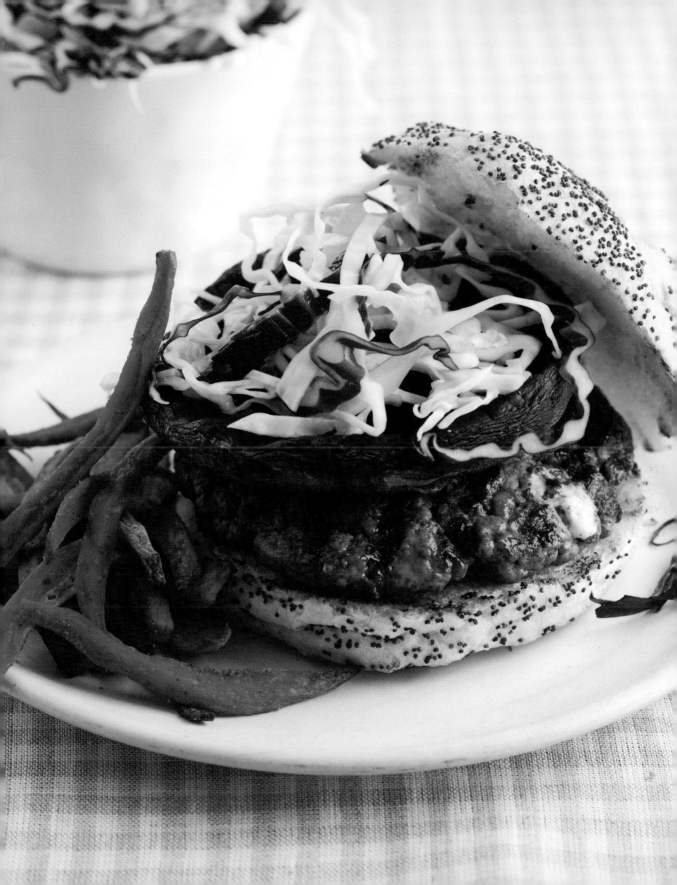

# Savory Mini-Meat Loaves
## Serves 8 to 10

This very easy recipe has a long list of ingredients, but it gives you some meat to enjoy while restricting fat and including fiber. The result is a reflux-friendly meat loaf—provided you eat only one! Because the taste and texture of ground turkey is not always optimal, I like to combine it with grass-fed beef, which contains only about one-sixth the saturated fat of ordinary ground beef. In addition to the meat, this recipe is chock full of fiber. Serve with steamed green beans or baby broccoli and $^1/_2$ cup per person of my Buttermilk Mashed Potatoes with Parsnips (page 171).

1 cup chopped yellow onion (about
    1 medium onion)

$^1/_2$ cup finely diced celery

2 tablespoons sunflower or canola oil

$^1/_2$ cup finely diced green bell pepper

2 cloves garlic, minced

1 pound ground turkey

1 pound lean ground beef, preferably grass-fed

1 cup rolled oats

2 eggs, lightly beaten

1 cup ketchup

2 tablespoons Dijon mustard

2 tablespoons Asian sesame oil

1 tablespoon Worcestershire sauce

1 teaspoon crushed cumin seed

1 teaspoon dried marjoram

1 cup cooked fresh or canned corn

$1^1/_2$ tablespoons soy sauce

In a medium skillet, combine the onion and celery with the sunflower oil. Cover and cook over medium heat for 3 to 5 minutes, until soft. Uncover and raise the heat to medium-high. Add the bell pepper and garlic and sauté for 3 to 5 minutes longer, until all the vegetables are soft and the onion is beginning to color. Remove from the heat and let cool to tepid.

Meanwhile, in a large bowl, combine the ground turkey and beef with the oats, eggs, $^1/_2$ cup of the ketchup, the mustard, 1 tablespoon of the sesame oil, the Worcestershire sauce, cumin seed, marjoram, and corn. Mix with your hands or a wooden spoon to blend well. Add the cooled onion mixture and blend well.

Preheat the oven to 375°F. Form the meat loaf mixture into 8 to 10 individual oval loaves about $4^1/_2$ inches long and $2^1/_2$ inches wide and arrange them on a baking sheet. (Line the sheet with foil for easy cleanup, if you like.)

In a small bowl, stir together the remaining $^1/_2$ cup ketchup and 1 tablespoon sesame oil with the soy sauce. Paint the meat loaves with this glaze and bake for 25 minutes, or until the meat is cooked through but still moist. Serve one meat loaf per person. Save any leftovers for eating hot or cold in the next day or two, or freeze for longer storage.

# Chapter 12

# PASTA, RICE, AND BEANS

# Orrechiette with Broccoli Rabe, Ricotta, and Sausage

Serves 6

Just a tiny bit of sausage adds a disproportionate amount of flavor here. Choose sweet or hot, depending upon your tolerance. But notice each person is getting only 1 ounce of that sausage, and as much fat as possible is extracted before it's added to the sauce. The result is a rich, flavorful dish that won't keep you up all night.

6 ounces Italian sausage, sweet or hot

3 tablespoons plus 2 teaspoons olive oil

1 pound orrechiette, preferably imported

3 cloves garlic, thinly sliced

1 large bunch broccoli rabe, cut into 1-inch pieces (about 2 pounds)

1 cup part-skim ricotta cheese

1/2 cup grated pecorino Romano cheese

Salt and freshly ground black pepper, or a pinch of red chile flakes, if you tolerate it

Remove the sausage from its casing and crumble into a medium nonstick skillet. Add 2 teaspoons of the olive oil and cook over medium heat, stirring, until the sausage is no longer pink and much of the fat has been rendered. Scrape the sausage into a sieve and drain off as much fat as possible, then blot on paper towels. Set aside on a plate.

In a large pot of boiling salted water, cook the orrechiette for 11 to 13 minutes, until it is tender but still firm; this pasta is thicker than most and takes a bit longer to cook. Scoop out and reserve 1/2 cup of the pasta cooking water. Drain the pasta into a colander.

In a large skillet or flameproof casserole, cook the garlic in the remaining 3 tablespoons olive oil over medium-high heat for 1 to 2 minutes, until fragrant but not brown. Add the broccoli rabe and cook, stirring, for 3 minutes longer. Add the reserved pasta cooking water, reduce the heat to medium, cover, and cook, stirring once or twice, for 4 to 5 minutes, until the broccoli rabe is tender but not mushy.

Add the cooked sausage, the ricotta, and the orrechiette. Stir gently to mix. Cover, reduce the heat to medium-low, and cook for about 2 minutes, until heated through. Toss with the pecorino Romano cheese, season with salt and pepper to taste, and serve.

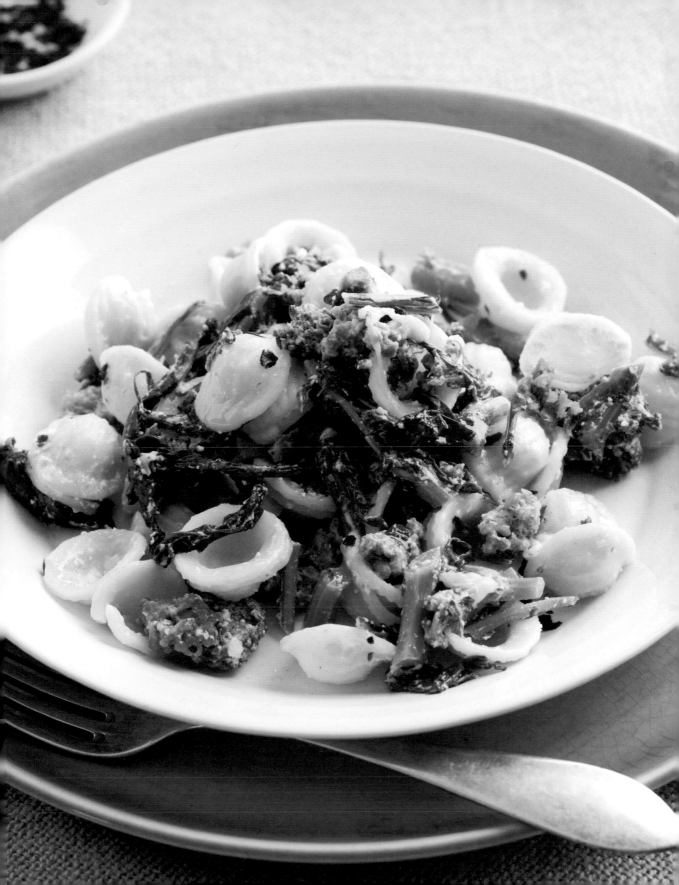

# Bowties with Roasted Cauliflower and Shiitakes

## Serves 4

I always pass grated cheese with this savory vegetarian pasta. If it's a nice snappy cheese, like pecorino Romano, it will perk up the mild cauliflower. And you'll need less cheese—and less fat—to fill out the taste. Or try a mix of grated Parmigiano-Reggiano and Manchego—not authentic, but delicious.

1 head cauliflower, separated into 1-inch florets

3 cloves garlic, slivered

2 teaspoons drained capers

$1/2$ teaspoon coarse salt

$1/4$ teaspoon Aleppo pepper (optional; see note)

$1/4$ cup extra virgin olive oil

4 ounces fresh shiitakes, stemmed and sliced

$1/2$ pound bowtie pasta

2 tablespoons mild red wine vinegar

3 tablespoons chopped fresh parsley

Preheat the oven to 425°F. In a 14-inch gratin dish or other shallow baking dish, combine the cauliflower, garlic, capers, salt, and Aleppo pepper. Drizzle on the olive oil and toss to coat. Pour $2/3$ cup water into the dish.

Roast the cauliflower for 10 minutes, stirring once. Add the shiitakes and roast for 15 minutes longer, stirring about halfway through.

Meanwhile, cook the pasta in 3 to 4 quarts of boiling salted water for 9 to 10 minutes, until just tender but still firm. Scoop out and reserve $1/2$ cup of the pasta cooking water. Drain the pasta into a colander.

Pour the pasta cooking water into the baking dish and use a wooden spoon to scrape up any browned bits. Sprinkle the vinegar and 2 tablespoons of the parsley over the vegetables. Add the pasta and toss to mix. Dust the top with the remaining 1 tablespoon parsley and serve.

NOTE: Aleppo pepper is a wonderful mildly hot pepper with good flavor, which makes a nice stand-in for the spicer varieties. If you think you cannot tolerate any heat at all, substitute freshly ground black peppercorns.

# Lemon-Pistachio Angel Hair

Serves 4 as a first course

Here's an exception to the reflux rule of eating as little saturated fat as possible. A little more cream than would normally be allowed but still a modest portion makes this a real treat to be enjoyed as a first course only. For simplicity, I buy my pistachios already shelled and roasted. Make the sauce, if you like, several hours in advance and toss with the pasta just before serving.

1 tablespoon minced shallot

1 tablespoon extra virgin olive oil

3 tablespoons dry vermouth

$1/2$ cup heavy cream

$1/3$ cup plus 1 tablespoon shelled and roasted pistachio nuts, finely chopped

Grated zest and juice from 1 small lemon

$1/8$ teaspoon freshly grated nutmeg

2 tablespoons chopped fresh parsley

Salt and freshly ground black pepper

5 to 6 ounces angel hair pasta

$1/3$ cup grated Parmigiano-Reggiano cheese

In a small saucepan, cook the shallot in the olive oil over medium heat for 1 to 2 minutes, until softened. Pour in the vermouth and cream. Add $1/3$ cup of the pistachios, the lemon zest, nutmeg, and 1 tablespoon of the parsley. Season to taste with salt and pepper. Bring to a boil, reduce the heat to low, and simmer for 5 minutes.

Cook the angel hair in $2^{1}/2$ to 3 quarts of boiling salted water for about 7 minutes, until just tender. Scoop out and reserve about $1/3$ cup of the cooking water. Drain the pasta.

Reheat the sauce, if necessary. Stir $1/4$ cup of the cheese and the lemon juice into the sauce. In a serving bowl, toss the pasta with the sauce. If it seems at all dry, add the reserved pasta cooking water, 1 tablespoon at a time. Sprinkle the remaining 1 tablespoon pistachios, $1^{1}/2$ tablespoons cheese, and 1 tablespoon parsley on top and serve.

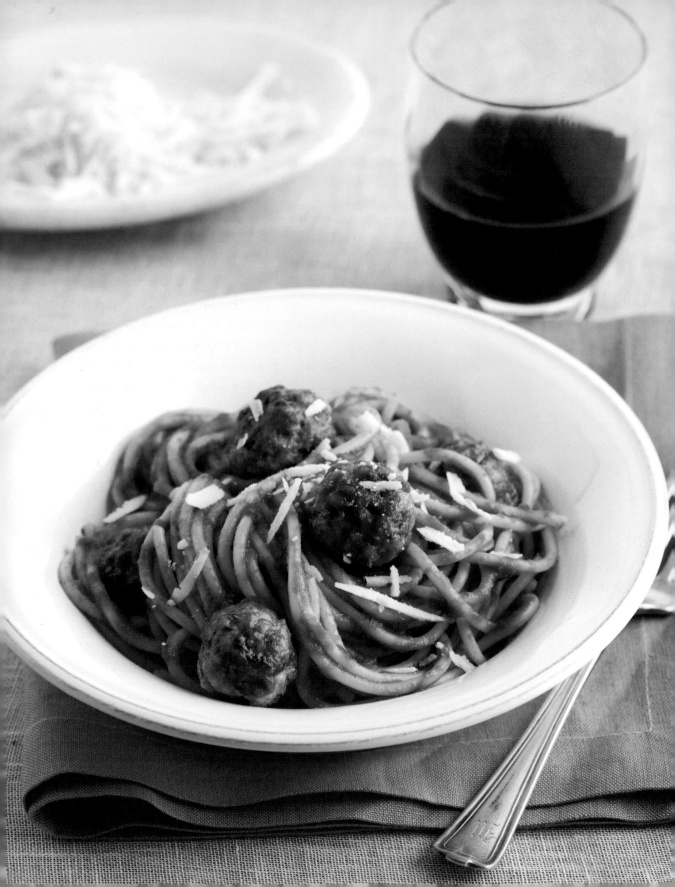

# Spaghetti and Meatballs

## Serves 6

Not with my GERD, you say? Well try this, just once, and see if you cannot go back to enjoying some of the comfort food you have always loved. The dish has been lightened in a number of ways. First of all, the tomato sauce is cut with chicken broth, and just enough is used to coat the pasta, not to bathe it. Secondly, the meatballs are lean, made with a blend of grass-fed beef and ground turkey, and they are broiled rather than fried. Notice: This recipe is designed to serve six. Enjoy a single portion, and you will be fine. Have seconds, and all bets are off.

1/2 cup finely chopped onion

1/2 cup finely chopped carrot

1/2 teaspoon demerara or turbinado sugar

1/2 teaspoon salt

3 tablespoons extra virgin olive oil

1 tablespoon tomato paste

1 cup Easy Rotisserie Chicken Stock (page 87), or any reduced-sodium chicken broth

1 (28-ounce) can diced tomatoes, preferably Pomi (see note, page 132)

1 (14-ounce) can strained tomatoes, preferably Pomi (see note, page 132)

Meatballs My Way (recipe follows)

1 pound spaghetti

Grated Parmigiano-Reggiano or pecorino Romano cheese

In a large pot, combine the onion, carrot, sugar, and salt with the olive oil. Sauté over medium-high heat for about 5 minutes, until golden and soft. Add the tomato paste and cook for 1 minute longer. Add the chicken broth and diced tomatoes, and simmer for 30 minutes. While the sauce is simmering, make the meatballs.

With an immersion blender, briefly puree the sauce until the tomatoes are finely chopped. Add the browned meatballs and simmer for 10 minutes.

In a large pot of boiling salted water, cook the spaghetti for about 10 minutes, until it is just barely al dente. Drain well.

Add the cooked spaghetti to the pot with the sauce and toss well. Partially cover and simmer over low heat for 2 to 3 minutes, until the pasta is just tender. Scoop into bowls and pass the grated cheese on the side.

*Continued*

## MEATBALLS MY WAY

Makes about 18 meatballs; serves 6

You'll be thrilled if you're lucky enough to have any of these left over. They make a great meatball sandwich. But be sure to use my vanishing roll technique (see page 142) if you do so. Ground meats are often sold labeled not by the amount of fat they contain, but by how lean they are. If you have a choice, choose ground beef that is anywhere from 96 to 98 percent lean, which is very lean, indeed, and ground turkey, which is about 94 percent lean. Notice that grass-fed beef contains less fat than turkey, and what it does contain has more "healthier" omega-3s, which the animal gets from the green grass it eats.

1 ounce firm-textured day-old white bread or Italian bread, crust removed

$1/4$ cup reduced-sodium chicken broth

1 egg

1 clove garlic, crushed through a press

$1/2$ teaspoon marjoram

$1/2$ teaspoon salt

$1/4$ teaspoon freshly grated nutmeg

$1/8$ teaspoon freshly ground black pepper

$1/4$ cup grated Parmigiano-Reggiano cheese

$1/4$ cup chopped fresh parsley

$1/2$ pound ground grass-fed beef (97 percent lean)

$1/2$ pound ground turkey (94 percent lean)

Preheat the broiler and place the oven rack about 4 inches from the heat. Lightly oil a baking sheet (lined with aluminum foil for easy cleanup, if you like).

Crumble the bread into coarse crumbs and place in a bowl. Add the chicken broth to the crumbs and let stand for 5 to 10 minutes, until completely moistened. Add the egg and garlic; beat with a fork to make a paste. Season with the marjoram, salt, nutmeg, and pepper. Add the cheese and parsley and blend well. Finally, add the ground beef and turkey and blend thoroughly with your hands.

Roll walnut-sized pieces of the ground meat mixture between your palms to make small meatballs about $1\frac{1}{4}$ inches in diameter; there will be about 18. Arrange on the prepared baking sheet about 1 inch apart. Broil the meatballs for 5 to 8 minutes, turning once about halfway through, until lightly browned on the outside. (Don't worry about the inside; the meatballs will finish cooking in the sauce.)

# Spaghettini with Broccolini
## Serves 4

Broccoli is one of those so-called cruciferous vegetables that have been associated with lower rates of several types of cancer. It is full of fiber, folate, calcium, and the important antioxidant vitamin C. Broccolini, which is sometimes billed as baby broccoli but is really a slightly different cultivar, is a sweeter form of the vegetable and holds its texture nicely even when tender. The trick of using some of the pasta cooking water in the sauce is authentically Italian.

1 large bunch Broccolini

Sea salt

1/2 pound spaghettini

2 1/2 tablespoons extra virgin olive oil

1 clove garlic, thinly sliced

1/4 teaspoon Aleppo pepper (optional; see note)

3 tablespoons finely diced sun-dried tomatoes

1/2 cup grated pecorino Romano cheese

Trim just the ends off the Broccolini and cut the stalks and florets into 1-inch lengths.

In a large saucepan, bring 3 quarts water with 1 tablespoon sea salt to a boil over high heat. Add the spaghettini, broken in half if you like, and cook for 7 to 9 minutes, until it is just al dente. Scoop out and reserve 1 cup of the cooking water. Drain the pasta into a colander and toss with 1/2 tablespoon of the olive oil so it doesn't stick together.

Wipe out the saucepan and return it to medium heat. Add the remaining 2 tablespoons olive oil, the garlic, and the Aleppo pepper. Cook for 1 to 2 minutes, until the garlic is softened and fragrant. Add the Broccolini pieces and the sun-dried tomatoes and stir to coat with the oil. Pour in the reserved pasta cooking water and cook for 4 to 5 minutes, until the Broccolini is just tender but still bright green.

Add the pasta and toss over the heat to mix well. Cover and cook over low heat for 1 to 2 minutes, until heated through. Toss with the cheese and serve.

NOTE: Aleppo pepper is a wonderful mildly hot pepper with good flavor, which makes a nice stand-in for the spicer varieties. If you think you cannot tolerate any heat at all, substitute freshly ground black peppercorns.

# Penne with Zucchini and Mushrooms

### Serves 4

I've softened the tomatoes here with stock and soy milk, which contains calcium, a base, to balance out the acid in the tomatoes. A mild, pink sauce results. Tender young zucchini and meaty mushrooms add plenty of fiber and nutrients and very few calories. I like a short, tubular pasta, such as pennette or mezze penne, to match the size of the zucchini and mushroom pieces. Plus, the smaller the pasta, the more you get in a single serving. One trick that's very Italian and produces a more flavorful dish with better texture is to undercook the pasta, then add it to the sauce and simmer for a few minutes. The pasta becomes saturated with the sauce while it turns just slightly al dente.

4 small zucchini (about 1 pound total)

8 ounces white mushrooms

Salt and freshly ground black pepper

3 tablespoons extra virgin olive oil

1 pound Roma tomatoes, peeled and seeded, or 1 (15-ounce) can diced peeled tomatoes

3 cloves garlic, sliced

2 tablespoons coarsely chopped fresh basil, or $1/2$ teaspoon dried thyme

1 tablespoon tomato paste

$1 1/4$ cups Easy Rotisserie Chicken Stock (page 87), any reduced-sodium chicken broth, or vegetable stock

$1/2$ cup enriched organic soy milk (see note)

$3/4$ pound pennette or mezze penne

$1/4$ cup grated pecorino Romano cheese, plus more for sprinkling

Preheat the broiler. Trim the ends off the zucchini. Cut them in half lengthwise, then cut crosswise into $1/2$-inch pieces. Trim the ends off the mushroom stems and then cut the mushrooms into quarters.

Place the zucchini and mushrooms in a bowl. Season lightly with salt and pepper, add 1 tablespoon of the olive oil, and toss to coat. Spread out the vegetables on a baking sheet and broil as close to the heat as possible, stirring once, for 8 minutes, or until the zucchini are beginning to brown but remain firm-tender. Remove and set aside.

Put the tomatoes and any juices into a food processor. Turn on the machine, and one at a time, drop the garlic cloves through the feed tube. Add the basil and process until finely chopped.

In a deep saucepan, heat the remaining 2 tablespoons olive oil over medium heat. Add the tomato paste and cook, stirring, for 2 to 3 minutes, until it darkens. Pour in the pureed tomatoes. Add the stock and soy milk. Season with salt and pepper to taste. Bring to a boil, reduce the heat to medium, and boil gently for 15 minutes. Remove from the heat.

In a large pot of boiling salted water, cook the pasta for 6 to 7 minutes, until it is not yet quite done. Drain into a colander. Return the pasta to the pot and add the tomato sauce. Simmer over low heat, stirring occasionally, for 2 to 3 minutes, until the pasta is just al dente. Add the ¼ cup cheese and the broiled vegetables and stir to mix. Pass a little extra cheese on the side.

NOTE: For best flavor, choose a neutral soy milk that does not have added sugar or vanilla flavoring, such as organic Eden brand.

# Butternut Squash Risotto

## Serves 6

Much less butter and more vegetables make this risotto less than traditional but much more GERD friendly. Enjoy a small portion as a first course before a dinner of simple chicken or fish and vegetables or indulge as a main dish for lunch with a green salad on the side. The quality of the stock makes a big difference with risotto, so if you've made any of my Easy Rotisserie Chicken Stock (page 87), now's the time to use it.

1 butternut squash, preferably organic (1$\frac{1}{4}$ to 1$\frac{1}{2}$ pounds)

1 yellow onion, chopped

2 tablespoons extra virgin olive oil

1 small fennel bulb, or 2 celery ribs, chopped

1 cup Arborio or other risotto rice

3 to 3$\frac{1}{4}$ cups Easy Rotisserie Chicken Stock (page 87), or any reduced-sodium chicken broth

1 teaspoon salt

$\frac{1}{2}$ teaspoon chopped fresh sage or crumbled dried

$\frac{1}{4}$ teaspoon freshly grated nutmeg

2 tablespoons unsalted butter

$\frac{2}{3}$ cup finely grated Parmigiano-Reggiano cheese

Preheat the oven to 400°F. Prick the squash in several places with the tip of a knife. Place in a small baking dish or pie plate and roast in the oven, turning once or twice, for 50 to 60 minutes, until the squash is soft and the skin is starting to brown. Slit the squash lengthwise and let cool. When it is cool enough to handle, peel off the skin, scoop out the seeds and any strings, and cut the squash into large chunks. In a large heavy pot, stir the onion into the olive oil over medium heat. Cover and cook for 3 to 5 minutes, until the onion is soft and translucent. Stir in the fennel, cover, and cook for 3 minutes longer. Uncover, raise the heat to medium-high, and cook, stirring occasionally, for 5 to 7 minutes, until the fennel is soft and the onion is golden and beginning to brown.

Add the rice. Cook, stirring, for 2 to 3 minutes, until the rice turns opaque. Pour in 1 cup of the stock. Add the salt, sage, and nutmeg. Cook, stirring, for about 3 minutes, until most of the stock is absorbed. Stir in another 1 cup of the stock and add the squash, stirring to blend it with the rice. Add another 1 cup stock, reduce the heat to medium, cover, and cook, stirring once or twice, for 15 minutes, or until the liquid is mostly absorbed and the rice is tender but still firm. If it seems too dry, add the remaining $\frac{1}{4}$ cup stock.

Stir in the butter until melted. Then add the cheese. Season with additional salt to taste and serve.

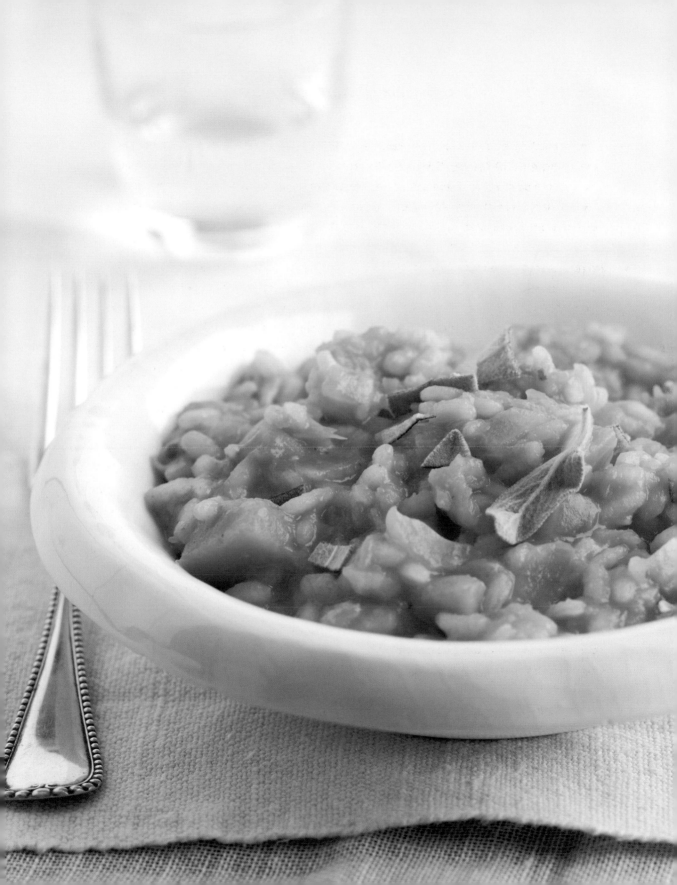

# Double Mushroom Risotto

## Serves 4

Rice is very easy to digest, so risotto is an excellent choice for anyone suffering from acid reflux. The only drawback is that the rice is normally swimming in butter and cheese, and the dish tastes so good, it's hard to stop eating. Well, as for portion control, we already know that mantra: If you want to avoid reflux, you simply must not eat too much at any one time. But we did devise a version with about one-third the normal butter and half the cheese that's much easier on the stomach.

You'll notice that there's an optional teaspoon and a half of truffle oil stirred in just before serving. If you have it, use it! Too many people squirrel away a bottle up on the top shelf of the cupboard, stowed away because it's so expensive. That's a mistake, because truffle oil is highly perishable—good for a year at most. Even if the oil doesn't become rancid, the truffle flavor fades. Just a tiny amount delivers a huge payoff in taste.

1 ounce dried porcini mushrooms

12 ounces white mushrooms

2 tablespoons olive oil

1 shallot, minced

1 cup Arborio or other risotto rice

2 tablespoons dry Marsala or Madeira

3 to 3$^1$/$_2$ cups Easy Rotisserie Chicken Stock (page 87), or any reduced-sodium chicken broth, heated

$^1$/$_2$ teaspoon dried thyme

$^1$/$_4$ teaspoon freshly ground nutmeg

2 tablespoons unsalted butter

1$^1$/$_2$ teaspoons white truffle oil (optional but luscious)

6 tablespoons grated cheese, preferably half Parmigiano-Reggiano and half pecorino Romano cheese

Salt and freshly ground black pepper

Soak the porcini in a bowl of hot water to cover for 20 to 30 minutes, until softened. Lift out the mushrooms and squeeze them dry, letting the excess liquid drip back into the bowl. Strain the liquid through a fine-mesh sieve or coffee filter to remove any grit.

Trim the ends off the white mushrooms. Thinly slice about one-fourth of them. Quarter the remainder, place in a food processor, and pulse until finely chopped.

Heat the olive oil in a heavy saucepan or flameproof casserole over medium-high heat. Add the shallot and cook, stirring, for 1 minute. Add the sliced mushrooms and cook, stirring occasionally, for about 5 minutes, until they begin to give up their liquid.

Add the rice and stir to coat. Cook, stirring, for 1 minute. Stir in the chopped mushrooms, then pour in the Marsala and let it cook away. Add ¾ cup of the simmering stock, the thyme, and the nutmeg. Cook, stirring, for 3 to 5 minutes, until the liquid evaporates. Add another cup of stock and continue to cook, stirring often and reducing the heat slightly if the liquid boils off too fast, until most of the stock is absorbed. Repeat with 1 cup stock until the rice is tender and only a little liquid remains. This usually takes about 18 minutes. If it seems too dry, add the remaining ½ cup stock.

Remove from the heat and add the butter and truffle oil, if you have it, and stir until the butter melts. Stir in ¼ cup of the cheese and season with salt and pepper to taste. Serve on plates or in shallow bowls, with the remaining 2 tablespoons cheese sprinkled on top.

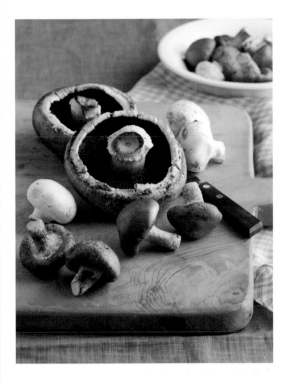

# Black Bean and Grilled Vegetable Chili

## Serves 6

Chili is normally a no-no for GERD sufferers, but there is no proven connection between spicy food and acid reflux. It's not clear whether spices really do act as a trigger in susceptible individuals, or whether we're just tempted to eat too much when food is robustly seasoned. If you do not have an inflamed throat, there is no reason you cannot enjoy this light, chunky chili with no saturated fat or tomatoes. Your only problem will be turning down seconds. For each serving, allow $1/2$ cup cooked brown rice to accompany the chili.

2 medium-large zucchini, cut lengthwise into
   3 long slices

2 long, thin Asian eggplants, halved

1 red bell pepper

1 large portobello mushroom cap

$1/3$ cup extra virgin olive oil

1 small onion, coarsely chopped

$3/4$ teaspoon demerara or turbinado sugar

2 cloves garlic, thinly sliced

1 to $1^1/2$ tablespoons ancho chile or other mild
   chile powder

2 teaspoons ground cumin

1 teaspoon dried oregano

$1/4$ teaspoon ground allspice

1 tablespoon vegetable bouillon powder

1 tablespoon cornmeal

2 (15-ounce) cans pinto or black beans, preferably
   organic, rinsed and drained

$3/4$ cup fresh or canned corn

Salt and freshly ground black pepper

Brush the zucchini, eggplants, bell pepper, and mushroom with 2 to 3 tablespoons of the olive oil. Grill over a hot fire or broil 3 to 4 inches from the heat, turning and rotating, until the zucchini and eggplants are just barely tender, about 3 minutes; the outside of the bell pepper is charred, about 5 minutes; and the mushroom is nicely browned and just barely softened, 5 to 7 minutes. Remove the vegetables as they are done and let cool. When you can handle them, cut the zucchini and eggplants crosswise into $1/2$-inch pieces. Peel the bell pepper and cut into $1/2$-inch squares. Cut the mushroom into $1/2$-inch dice.

In a large flameproof casserole, cook the onion with the sugar in the remaining $2^1/2$ to $3^1/2$ tablespoons olive oil over medium heat for about 5 minutes, until the onion is softened and golden. Add the garlic, chile powder, cumin, and oregano. Cook for 2 minutes longer to toast the spices. Pour in 4 cups water and bring to a boil. Stir in the allspice and bouillon powder. Return to a boil; reduce the heat to a simmer.

Sprinkle the cornmeal over the liquid in the casserole and stir in. Bring to a boil, stirring. Add all the vegetables to the sauce base, reduce the heat, and simmer for 5 minutes. Add the beans and corn and simmer for 10 minutes. Season with salt and pepper to taste.

# Beans and Greens

## Serves 4

Beans go both ways: They're good for you because they're exceptionally rich in fiber and offer a virtually fat-free source of protein. In addition, they contain iron, folate, and other B vitamins as well as calcium. On the other hand, as we all know, they can cause a build-up of pressure from gas, which can bring on reflux. Over-the-counter aids, like Bean-O, are only partially effective and do not work for everyone. The best advice is to eat beans with restraint, which means 1/2 cup, an amount most people can deal with easily. Enjoy this dish as a vegetarian stew all by itself or use it as a sauce over pasta or rice.

1 small leek, white and tender green parts,
    or 1 large shallot, thinly sliced

1 1/2 tablespoons extra virgin olive oil

1 bunch lacinato kale, stemmed and coarsely
    shredded (8 cups)

1 cup Easy Rotisserie Chicken Stock (page 87), or
    any reduced-sodium chicken broth, vegetable
    stock, or bean cooking broth if you've made
    your own

2 cups Best Pot of Beans (made with cranberry or
    cannellini beans; page 162) or canned beans,
    preferably organic, rinsed and drained

Salt and freshly ground black pepper or Aleppo
    pepper (see note)

In a large skillet or flameproof casserole, cook the leek in the olive oil over medium heat for 3 to 5 minutes, until softened.

Raise the heat to medium-high and add the kale, in batches, stirring, until it wilts slightly. Add the stock, reduce the heat to medium-low, cover partially, and cook for 7 to 10 minutes, until the kale is tender but still bright green.

Add the beans and fold to mix them with the greens. Season with salt and pepper to taste. Simmer for 5 minutes longer.

NOTE: Aleppo pepper is a wonderful mildly hot pepper with good flavor, which makes a nice stand-in for the spicer varieties. If you think you cannot tolerate any heat at all, substitute freshly ground black peppercorns.

# Best Pot of Beans

Makes 4 to 5 cups; serves 6 to 8

If you're making chili for a crowd, you could double the recipe, but half a pound of dried beans makes plenty for just about any purpose you choose to use them: in a salad, as a side dish, or baked. The recipe below is my favorite basic formula. If heat doesn't bother you, toss in 1 dried smoked serrano or chipotle chile. If you have them on hand, also add a few parsley or thyme sprigs.

$1/2$ pound dried beans (about 1 cup), preferably organic

1 yellow onion

2 whole cloves

1 celery rib with leaves

3 cloves garlic, cut in half

1 bay leaf

Soak the beans overnight in a bowl with enough water to cover by at least 2 inches.

Drain the beans and put them in a $3^{1}/_{2}$- to 4-cup pot. Halve the onion and stick a clove into each piece; add to the pot. Add the celery, garlic, and bay leaf. Pour in enough cold water to cover the beans by about $1/2$ inch.

Bring to a simmer, reduce the heat to medium-low, and cook, partially covered, for 45 to 50 minutes, until the beans are tender but still firm. If the liquid gets too low, add more, $1/2$ cup at a time.

Remove from the heat, cover, and let stand for 10 to 15 minutes. Pick out and discard the bay leaf and aromatics. Drain the beans, reserving the pot liquid for soup stock, if you like.

NOTE: After cooking, I like to salt the beans and toss them with just a little extra virgin olive oil. Refrigerate in a covered container for up to 5 days. Use them in salads, stews, soups, or mixed with rice for a vegetarian main course.

# Chapter 13

# VEGETABLES AND GRAINS

# Asparagus with Orange-Olive Dressing

## Serves 4

Steamed asparagus in season with just a drizzle of olive oil is heavenly. A highly alkaline vegetable, it contributes potassium, calcium, and vitamin A. Add to it these hits of Mediterranean flavor, and you've got a snappy vegetable fine enough to serve as a starter, or a bright accompaniment to a simple chicken or fish, such as our Asian Barbecued Chicken (page 128). If you are one of those reflux sufferers who must avoid citrus, don't dismiss this recipe. A smidgeon of grated zest and a couple of tablespoons of juice are a far cry from a glass of orange juice—I promise you.

1 pound fresh asparagus, preferably in season

$^1/_2$ teaspoon grated zest plus 2 tablespoons fresh juice from 1 orange

1 tablespoon walnut oil or extra virgin olive oil

$^1/_8$ teaspoon freshly ground black pepper

2 tablespoons minced pitted kalamata olives

2 tablespoons chopped walnuts

Trim the asparagus to 7 to 8 inches, just small enough to fit in your pot. Steam on a rack over boiling water for 3 to 4 minutes, until the asparagus is just tender but still bright green. Transfer to a platter.

In a small bowl, whisk together the orange zest and juice, walnut oil, and pepper. Stir in the olives and walnuts. Pour over the asparagus and turn gently with tongs to coat with the dressing. Serve warm or at room temperature.

# Balsamic Beets

Makes 1$\frac{1}{2}$ to 2 cups; serves 4

Beets are not only colorful and delicious, but they are also full of antioxidants and contain a chemical, called betaine, that can help prevent anemia if you're not absorbing enough B$_{12}$. Granted, you'd probably have to eat an awful lot of beets to do the trick. I often make a double batch of this recipe, which is more of a condiment than a vegetable, and keep it on hand to throw into salads or brighten up a dull plate. These are what I always use for the Gingered Beet and Scallop Salad on page 107.

1 bunch fresh beets

1 tablespoon balsamic vinegar

$\frac{1}{2}$ teaspoon ground coriander seed

Preheat the oven to 400°F.

Cut the stems off the beets, leaving about 1 inch as well as the thin roots attached. Rinse the beets well and wrap in a double layer of aluminum foil so they don't leak. Roast in the oven for 45 to 55 minutes, until you can slide a knife in easily.

Remove and let cool in their wrapping. When cool enough to handle, peel the beets; the skins should slip right off.

Cut the beets into $\frac{1}{2}$-inch dice. Toss with the vinegar and coriander. Refrigerate in a covered container for up to 5 days.

# Ginger-Glazed Carrots with Cauliflower and Snow Peas

### Serves 4 to 6

A steamer makes vegetable cooking quick and easy and conserves both nutrients and energy while enhancing color and flavor. This simple tricolor side dish, packed with fiber and vitamins, goes well with almost any meat, chicken, or fish, such as our Rosemary-Fennel Chicken Cutlets (page 134) or Shrimp-Stuffed Tilapia (page 123).

4 medium carrots, peeled and cut into
   $3/4$-inch pieces

1 pound cauliflower, cut into 1-inch florets

4 ounces snow peas, ends trimmed

1 tablespoon minced fresh ginger

$1/2$ shallot, minced

$1^1/2$ tablespoons extra virgin olive oil

1 teaspoon demerara or turbinado sugar

$1/4$ teaspoon ground ginger

In a steamer over about $1^1/2$ inches boiling water, cook the carrots for 4 minutes. Add the cauliflower to the pot and cook for 3 to 4 minutes, until the cauliflower is almost fully tender. Add the snow peas and steam for 2 minutes longer, until bright green but still slightly crisp.

In a large skillet, sauté the fresh ginger and shallot in the olive oil over medium-high heat for about 2 minutes, until fragrant. Sprinkle on the sugar and ground ginger. Add all the steamed vegetables and toss for about 2 minutes, until coated and heated through.

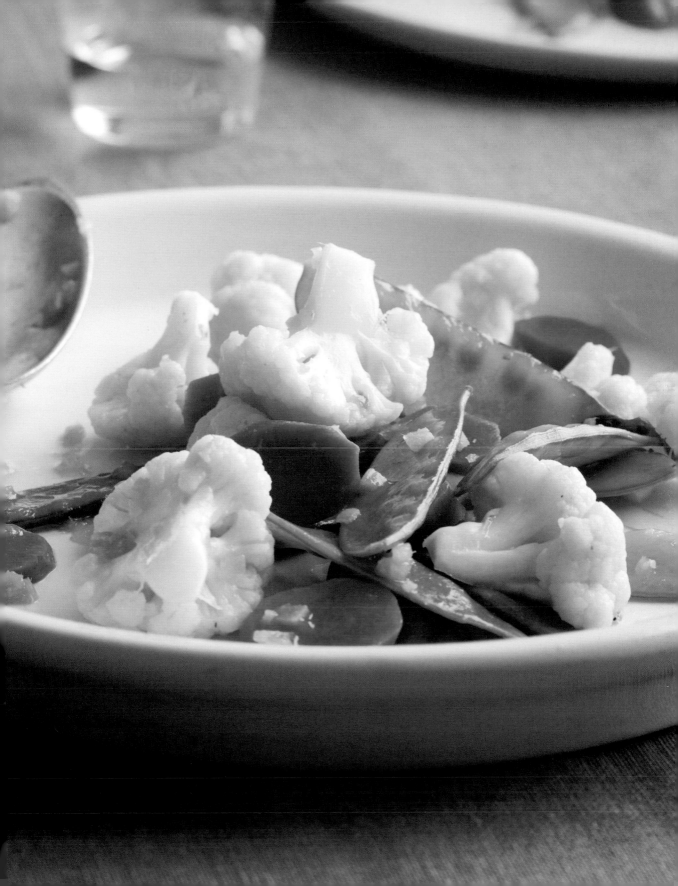

# Whipped Cauliflower with Parmesan Cheese

## Serves 4

Before you add any fat or liquid, about $2/3$ cup mashed potatoes has roughly 75 calories; the same amount of cauliflower has 25 at most. Don't tell anyone, and they'll think they are eating mashed potatoes—at a small fraction of the calories and with lots more nutrition. This is a mild, light dish that can accompany anything from Crispy Braised Chicken with Smoked Paprika (page 129) to Pistachio-Crusted Salmon with Braised Cabbage (page 119). The white truffle oil is extravagant, but worth it for the flavor.

1 medium-large head cauliflower (about $1^1/2$ pounds)

2 tablespoons unsalted butter

2 tablespoons grated Parmigiano-Reggiano cheese (optional)

1 teaspoon white truffle or olive oil, or
$1^1/2$ teaspoons additional unsalted butter

$3/8$ teaspoon sea salt

Dash of cayenne pepper (optional)

Cut the cauliflower into large florets. Steam for 12 to 15 minutes, until very soft. Transfer to a bowl.

Add the butter, cheese, truffle oil, sea salt, and cayenne. Beat with an electric mixer until completely smooth, light, and fluffy. You can puree the cauliflower in a food processor, but the texture will not be as airy.

# Ratatouille with Grilled Eggplant

## Serves 6

Ratatouille can be problematic for some, because even though it's made with healthful olive oil, many recipes use so much to sauté the eggplant that the dish turns out too greasy to be easily digestible. Here, the eggplant is grilled first with just a lick of oil; an entire portion contributes less than 2 teaspoons a person. Because this dish is so flavorful, it provides a good foil for simple meats, such as the Herb-Crusted Rack of Lamb with Savory White Beans (page 140) or Baked Flounder over Fennel Niçoise (page 113).

2 medium eggplants, 3/4 to 1 pound each

3 tablespoons extra virgin olive oil

1/2 red onion

3/4 teaspoon demerara or turbinado sugar

1/2 teaspoon salt

2 cloves garlic, minced

1 1/2 tablespoons tomato paste

2 Roma tomatoes or 4 small plum tomatoes, peeled, seeded, and diced

1 small red bell pepper, cut into 1/2-inch dice

2 medium zucchini, halved lengthwise, then sliced crosswise

3/4 teaspoon ground coriander

Freshly ground black pepper

Peel just 2 opposite sides of the eggplants. Then cut the vegetable lengthwise into 1/2- to 3/4-inch slices. (Each slice will have a ribbon of dark peel around the edge.) Brush the slices lightly with about 1 tablespoon of the olive oil. Grill over a medium-hot fire in a barbecue grill or on a cast iron stovetop grill pan, turning once, for about 5 minutes, until nicely browned outside but still fairly firm; the eggplants will finish cooking later.

In a large flameproof casserole, heat 1 1/2 tablespoons of the olive oil over medium-high heat. Add the red onion and sprinkle with the sugar and salt. Cook, stirring occasionally, for 3 to 4 minutes, until the onion is soft and beginning to color at the edges. Add the garlic and cook for 1 minute longer. Add the tomato paste and sauté for about 2 minutes, until it darkens slightly.

Add the tomatoes, bell pepper, zucchini, and coriander. Stir to mix everything well. Cover the pot, reduce the heat to medium, and simmer, stirring occasionally, for 5 to 7 minutes, until the zucchini is barely tender.

Meanwhile, dice the grilled eggplants. Add the eggplants to the casserole and fold to incorporate. Reduce the heat to medium-low and simmer for 5 to 7 minutes longer, until all the vegetables are tender and the flavors have blended.

If you have time, let the dish stand at room temperature for an hour or so, then reheat. Just before serving, stir in the remaining 1 1/2 teaspoons olive oil and season generously with pepper.

# Skillet-Braised Fennel

## Serves 4

Fennel is reputed to enhance digestion, so here's a double dose: the fresh bulb as well as fennel seeds. Cooked until it's almost caramelized and sweet, it's light and enticing. This fiber-rich vegetable goes beautifully with chicken and seafood. It would make a marvelous accompaniment for the Asian Barbecued Chicken (page 128) or as a substitute for cabbage with the Pistachio-Crusted Salmon (page 119). Fennel browns well in a cast iron or other heavy skillet.

1 1/2 to 2 fresh fennel bulbs

1/4 red onion

2 tablespoons extra virgin olive oil

1/2 teaspoon fennel seed, crushed

1/2 teaspoon demerara or turbinado sugar

1/4 teaspoon sea salt

1 cup Easy Rotisserie Chicken Stock (page 87), or any reduced-sodium chicken broth

Thickly slice the fennel and cut enough into roughly 1/2-inch dice to measure 3 1/2 to 4 cups. Thinly slice the red onion, then cut crosswise into 1/2-inch pieces.

In a large heavy skillet, preferably cast iron, cook the red onion in the olive oil over medium-high heat for 1 minute. Add the fresh fennel and season with the fennel seed, sugar, and salt. Cook for 3 to 5 minutes, tossing with the oil and turning with a spatula, until some pieces begin to brown.

Add the stock, cover, and reduce the heat to medium-low. Simmer for 10 minutes, stirring once or twice, until the fennel is soft. Uncover and if there is extra liquid remaining in the skillet, simmer for a couple of minutes until the vegetables are just moist.

# Buttermilk Mashed Potatoes with Parsnips

## Serves 4 to 6

While it is true that mashed potatoes do not have the lowest glycemic index, they are a particularly good source of potassium and should not be ignored. Nutty buttermilk, which despite its name is actually low in fat, and just a touch of real butter along with the sweetness of the parsnips make a special puree, indeed. These yummy but eminently digestible potatoes are the perfect accompaniment for the Savory Mini–Meat Loaves (page 144) or the Salmon Filet Mignon with Herb Butter (page 122).

1 1/2 pounds Yukon gold potatoes, peeled and cut into chunks

1/2 pound parsnips, peeled and sliced

2 tablespoons unsalted butter

1/2 cup low-fat buttermilk

1/2 teaspoon salt

1/8 teaspoon freshly ground black pepper

1/4 teaspoon freshly grated nutmeg

Boil the potatoes and the parsnips in a large pot of boiling salted water for 20 to 25 minutes, until tender. Scoop out and reserve 1/2 cup of the cooking water, then drain the vegetables. Put the potatoes and parsnips through a ricer or food mill or mash by hand. (Do not use a food processor, or they might turn gluey.)

Add the butter and stir until melted. Stir in the buttermilk. If the puree is too thick, add a little of the reserved cooking water, 2 tablespoons at a time. Season with the salt, pepper, and nutmeg.

# Braised Kale with Currants and Pine Nuts

### Serves 4

If you're taking proton pump inhibitors (PPIs), it's essential to make sure you're getting enough calcium and iron. Long-term use of PPIs is strongly associated with osteoporosis and iron-deficiency anemia. Vegetables like kale, spinach, collards, and broccoli rabe are good fat-free sources of calcium, iron, and folate—all important for combatting the effects of the drugs. The reason PPIs block absorption is that they prevent secretion of stomach acid, and minerals cannot enter the gut without some acid. That's why the recipe includes just enough lemon juice to enhance intake.

1 pound lacinato kale

2 cloves garlic, chopped

2 tablespoons extra virgin olive oil

1/4 cup currants

1/2 cup reduced-sodium chicken broth, vegetable stock, or water

3 tablespoons pine nuts, toasted (see note)

1 tablespoon balsamic vinegar

1 1/2 teaspoons freshly squeezed lemon juice

Salt and freshly ground black pepper

Trim the thick stems off the kale and cut the leaves crosswise into strips. In a large skillet or flameproof casserole, cook the garlic in the olive oil over medium heat for about 2 minutes, until softened and fragrant.

Add the kale, in batches if necessary, turning it as it wilts so it all fits into the pot. Add the currants and pour in the broth. Cover, reduce the heat to medium-low, and simmer, stirring occasionally, for 7 to 10 minutes, until the kale is just tender but still a nice green.

If more than a couple of tablespoons of liquid remain on the bottom of the pan, cook uncovered for a few minutes to evaporate. Toss the braised kale with the pine nuts, vinegar, and lemon juice. Season with salt and pepper to taste.

NOTE: Place a small skillet over medium heat. Add the pine nuts and toast, shaking the pan often, for 3 to 5 minutes, until the nuts are lightly browned and fragrant.

# Frizzled Kale

Serves 4

It's unbelievable how fast this technique turns tough, ordinary kale into a gossamer light treat. A cross between a garnish and a vegetable, the frizzled kale has a pleasing crispness and irresistible nutty flavor. Be sure to watch carefully while the kale cooks, because it can go from perfectly crisp to incinerated in just a couple of minutes. Choose grapeseed or refined canola cooking spray here to withstand the high-temperature cooking.

1 large bunch curly kale

Nonstick vegetable oil cooking spray, preferably grapeseed or refined canola

Sea salt

Preheat the oven to 400°F. Tear the kale leaves off the thick stems into 2½- to 3-inch pieces. Soak in a bowl of cold water, then spin as dry as possible.

Line a shallow baking sheet with aluminum foil for easy cleanup. Spread out the kale on the sheet. Shake the can of cooking spray well, then quickly spritz the kale. Turn the leaves over and spritz again briefly.

Toast the kale in the oven for 5 to 7 minutes, watching carefully, until crisp but still bright green. Season with a sprinkling of sea salt and serve at once.

# Spanish Potato Gratin

Serves 6 to 8

A bit lighter than the French gratin but richer than many of the recipes in this book, this Iberian version of the classic is a treat for when you absolutely crave something a little creamy. It makes a nice accompaniment to the Herb-Crusted Rack of Lamb (page 140) instead of the ragout of white beans.

1½ tablespoons unsalted butter, plus more for the pan

½ yellow onion, very thinly sliced

6 Yukon gold potatoes, peeled and thinly sliced about ⅛ inch thick

1 teaspoon smoked paprika, preferably pimentón de la Vera

Salt and freshly ground black pepper

1⅓ cups reduced-sodium chicken broth

½ cup half-and-half

1 cup shredded Idiazábal or Manchego cheese (about 3½ ounces)

Preheat the oven to 400°F. Butter a 14-inch oval flameproof gratin dish.

Line the bottom of the dish with the onion slices, spreading them out to cover evenly. Arrange the potato slices over the onion, overlapping slightly, in concentric circles like an apple tart. Begin at the edges and work in toward the center.

Sprinkle the smoked paprika over the potatoes and season with salt and pepper. Drizzle the chicken broth and half-and-half over the dish. Sprinkle the cheese over the top and dot with the butter.

Cover with aluminum foil and bring to a boil on top of the stove. Transfer to the oven and bake for 45 minutes. Uncover and bake for about 15 minutes longer, until most of the liquid is evaporated and the top is golden brown.

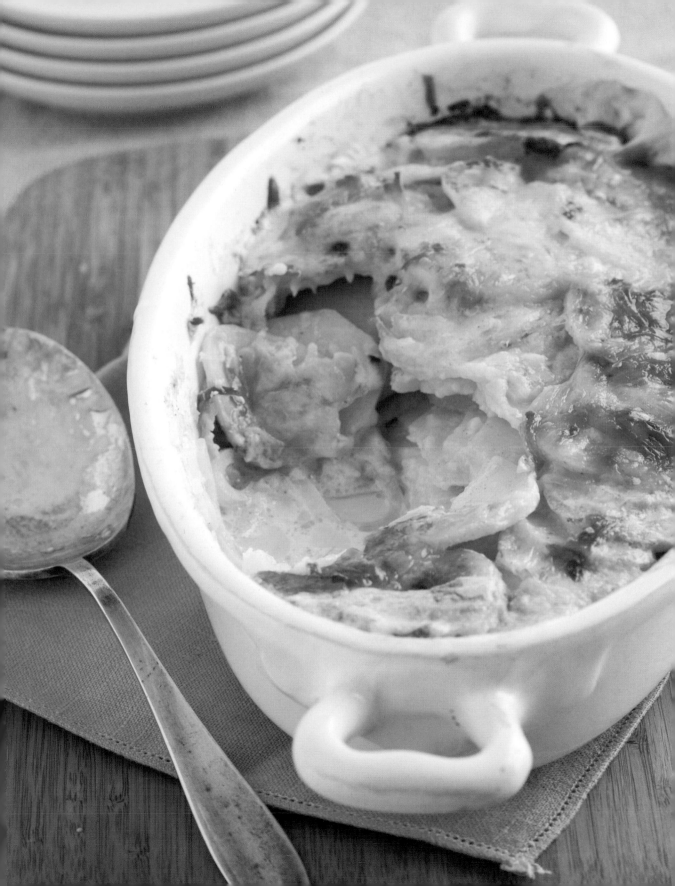

# Sesame Steamed Spinach

## Serves 2

It takes very little sesame oil to get a big hit of flavor. Tossing the spinach leaves in advance coats them easily and ensures even distribution. Don't be deceived by what looks like a lot of spinach; the leaves deflate hugely when cooked, so watch your timing carefully. To serve four, make two separate batches; it takes only a few minutes.

12 ounces prewashed baby spinach

2 teaspoons toasted sesame oil

$1/2$ teaspoon demerara or turbinado sugar

Salt and freshly ground black pepper

2 teaspoons toasted sesame seeds

Toss the spinach with the sesame oil, sugar, and salt and pepper to taste. Steam on a rack over boiling water for about 2 minutes, until the leaves are just wilted but still bright green.

Serve with the sesame seeds sprinkled on top.

# Gingered Sweet Potato Mash

Serves 4

Sweet potatoes seem mild and friendly, but they are nutrient powerhouses, full of beta-carotene, vitamin C, and fiber. While rich tasting, they are actually quite low in calories. Doubly laced with both candied and dried ginger, which is a traditional aid to digestion, this puree is irresistible and easily digestible. Serve with roast turkey or chicken, or as a component of a brightly colored vegetarian plate along with Balsamic Beets (page 165) and steamed zucchini or Asparagus with Orange-Olive Dressing (page 164).

2 pounds sweet potatoes

1 1/2 tablespoons sunflower oil

1 tablespoon unsalted butter

1 1/2 to 2 tablespoons finely diced glacéed ginger

1/2 teaspoon ground ginger

Preheat the oven to 400°F. Prick each sweet potato 2 or 3 times with the tip of a knife and put in a shallow baking dish. Roast for 40 to 45 minutes, until very soft.

As soon as the sweet potatoes are cool enough to handle, split in half and scoop into a bowl. Blend in the oil and butter. Stir in the glacéed and ground ginger.

# Baked Sweet Potato Fries

Serves 4

Even the thought of french fries makes my stomach gurgle; it also brings a smile to my face. I love them, but I can't eat them. When the issue is acid reflux, deep-fried food is out. Sad but true. Here's a low-fat—and low-calorie—substitute that I hope will take away some of your loss, as it does mine, while it alleviates your GERD. These are great with meaty dishes, such as our Grass-Fed Beef and Portobello Blue Cheese Burgers (page 142) or individual Savory Mini–Meat Loaves (page 144).

1½ pounds sweet potatoes

1½ tablespoons sunflower oil

1 teaspoon ground cumin

1 teaspoon turbinado or light brown sugar

¼ teaspoon salt

Preheat the oven to 425°F. Peel the sweet potatoes. Cut them lengthwise into ½-inch slices. Lay flat and cut into about ½-inch-thick strips that look like thick fries.

Put the sweet potato strips in a bowl. Drizzle on the oil and sprinkle with the cumin, sugar, and salt. Toss to coat evenly. Spread out the "fries" on a baking sheet (lined with aluminum foil for easy cleanup, if you like).

Bake for 15 to 20 minutes, until slightly browned and tender, carefully turning the strips about halfway through.

# Red Quinoa with Sesame and Currants

Serves 4 to 6

Quinoa is a wonderful grain with plenty of fiber, no gluten, and complete protein, just like soy. When cooking the grain, it's important to keep in mind the tiny seeds are covered with a bitter, naturally protective coating, called saponin. It takes literally seconds to remove by swishing the grain around in a bowl of warm water, but it makes all the difference in taste. Some companies are starting to sell prewashed quinoa. It's pricey but may be worth it to you.

1 cup red quinoa (see note)

2 teaspoons vegetable bouillon powder

1/2 cup dried currants

2 teaspoons toasted sesame oil

1 tablespoon chopped fresh parsley

Fill a medium bowl three-quarters full with warm water. Add the quinoa and swish it around with your fingers. Pour into a fine-mesh sieve and return to the bowl. Add more warm water, swish again, and drain.

In a small saucepan, bring 2²/₃ cups water to a boil with the bouillon powder. Add the quinoa and currants. Cover the pan, reduce the heat to low, and cook for 15 minutes, stirring. If there is still moisture at the bottom of the pot, cook, uncovered, for 5 minutes longer. You can tell when the quinoa is done because its little "tails" will unfurl.

Transfer to a bowl and toss with the sesame oil and parsley. Serve warm or at room temperature.

NOTE: The red variety is attractive and, I think, a tad sweeter, but regular quinoa is interchangeable here.

# DESSERTS

# Apple Coffee Cake

Makes a 9-inch square cake; serves 9

Just sweet enough for dessert, there is so much apple in this cake, you can enjoy it for breakfast as well. Whether dubbed an after-dinner pastry or a coffee cake, it's an any-time-of-day treat that's low in fat and rich in taste. But always keep in mind before you cut another piece: this recipe serves 9.

2 large Granny Smith or other baking apples

1 egg

2/3 cup packed light brown sugar

1 1/2 teaspoons vanilla extract

1/2 cup sunflower oil

1 1/3 cups all-purpose flour

1 teaspoon baking powder

1/2 teaspoon baking soda

1/4 teaspoon salt

2 teaspoons ground cinnamon

2/3 cup buttermilk

2 tablespoons demerara or turbinado sugar

Preheat the oven to 375°F. Lightly coat a 9-inch square baking pan with cooking spray. Peel and quarter the apples; cut out the stems and cores. Cut the apples into 1/2- to 3/4-inch chunks. In a large bowl, beat the egg, brown sugar, and vanilla. Gradually beat in the oil. In a separate bowl, mix together the flour, baking powder, baking soda, salt, and 1 teaspoon of the cinnamon. Add these dry ingredients to the batter, alternating with the buttermilk in 2 or 3 additions, stirring just until mixed.

Spread about one-quarter of the batter over the bottom of the baking pan. Add the apples to the remaining batter and fold to mix evenly. Turn into the baking pan. In a small bowl, stir together the demerara sugar and remaining 1 teaspoon cinnamon. Sprinkle over the top of the cake.

Bake for 30 to 35 minutes, until the cake is set throughout and just beginning to pull away from the sides of the pan. Let cool completely in the pan before cutting into 9 squares.

# Almond Polenta Cake

Makes an 8½-inch round cake; serves 8 to 10

Many people find highly refined carbohydrates backfire literally, so this tasty cake, which cuts the flour with ground almonds and polenta, may be a solution, especially if served in very thin slices. Serve the cake plain, with a dusting of confectioners' sugar, or dress it up with sliced fruit or berries and a small dollop of whipped cream or sweetened yogurt.

¾ cup finely ground polenta or stone-ground cornmeal

¾ cup unbleached all-purpose flour, preferably organic

¼ cup finely ground almond meal

2 teaspoons baking powder

3 extra-large eggs

⅔ cup demerara or turbinado sugar

1 teaspoon vanilla extract

¼ teaspoon almond extract

⅓ cup sunflower oil

3 tablespoons unsalted butter, melted and cooled slightly

Confectioners' sugar, for dusting (optional)

Sliced fruit or berries, for topping (optional)

Whipped cream or sweetened yogurt, for topping (optional)

Preheat the oven to 350°F. Lightly grease an 8½-inch springform pan. Line the bottom with a round of waxed paper and grease the paper.

In a small bowl, combine the polenta, flour, almond meal, and baking powder. Mix well.

In a separate bowl, beat the eggs with an electric mixer on medium speed. Add the sugar gradually and continue to beat for 3 to 4 minutes, until the eggs are lighter in color. Beat in the vanilla and almond extract.

Sprinkle about one-third of the dry ingredients over the egg mixture. Beat on low speed to barely blend. Drizzle on half the oil and beat briefly to mix. Sprinkle on half the remaining dry ingredients, drizzle on the remaining oil, and beat just until blended. Scrape down the sides of the bowl. Sprinkle on the remaining dry ingredients and the melted butter and beat until blended. Scrape the batter into the prepared springform pan.

Bake the cake for 35 minutes, or until the cake feels springy when touched lightly and a wooden toothpick inserted into the center comes out moist but clean. Do not wait until the cake pulls away from the sides of the pan, or it will be too dry.

Let stand for 10 minutes, then remove from the pan, transfer to a wire rack, and let cool before topping or serving.

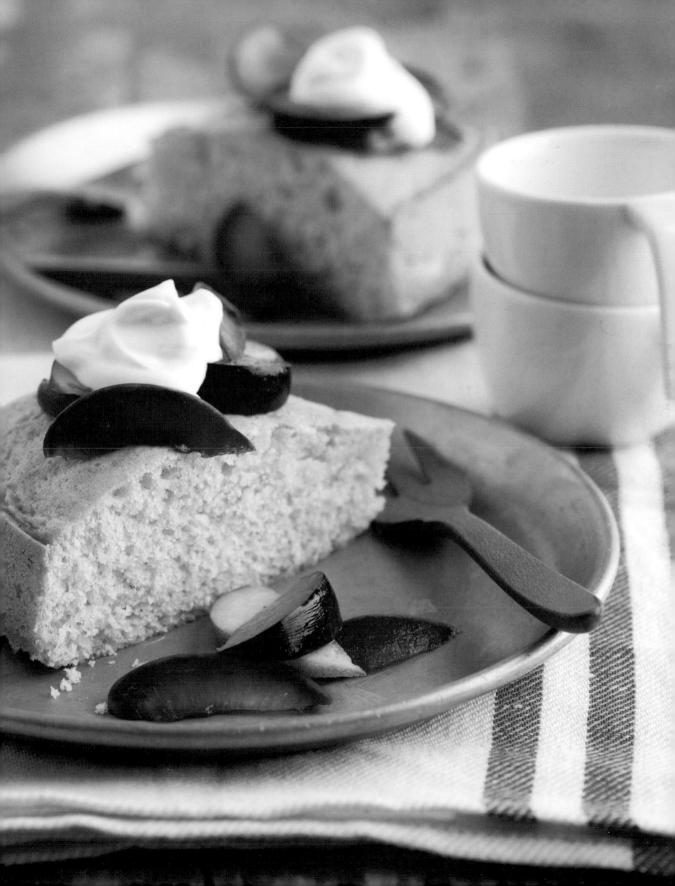

# Apple-Pear-Fig Turnovers

Makes 12 to 14 ($2^1/_2$-inch) turnovers; allow 2 per serving

Full of fiber and almost fat free, these delightful treats were created by Alisa Huntsman, the author of *Desserts from the Famous Loveless Cafe*. You can eat these warm, or bake them ahead and reheat the next day. They even freeze beautifully if you want to make a batch and ration them out.

1 medium-large Golden Delicious apple, peeled and cut into small dice

1 large ripe pear, preferably Bartlett or Anjou, peeled and cut into small dice

$1/_3$ cup dried Mission figs, stemmed and finely diced (6 to 8 figs)

$1/_4$ cup golden raisins

4 teaspoons brown rice flour

4 tablespoons organic cane sugar

$1/_2$ pound phyllo dough, thawed

Preheat the oven to 350°F. Line 2 cookie sheets with parchment or silicone sheets. Lightly coat with cooking spray.

In a bowl, combine the apple, pear, figs, raisins, brown rice flour, and 3 tablespoons of the sugar. Toss gently to mix. Set the fruit filling aside.

On a large cutting board, place a single sheet of phyllo dough. Give the dough a light spritz of cooking spray, top with a second sheet of dough, and spritz it. Repeat with a third sheet. Using a pizza cutter or large, sharp knife, cut the stack of dough in half lengthwise to make 2 long, thin stacks of dough. Dollop a heaping tablespoon of the fruit filling in one corner on the short side of each stack of dough. Just as you would fold up a flag, cover the fruit with the other corner and continue to fold the triangle back and forth until you reach the opposite end. Repeat with the rest of the dough sheets and filling.

Arrange the turnovers on the prepared baking sheets. Give them a light spritz of cooking spray and dust lightly with the remaining 1 tablespoon sugar.

Bake the fruit turnovers for about 25 minutes, until golden brown. Let cool for at least 10 to 15 minutes. Serve warm or at room temperature.

# Banana Pudding

Serves 6 to 8

Bananas are as soothing to the tummy as it gets. In fact, right after a patient has had sur-gery, I sometimes put them on what is called the BRAT diet: bananas, rice, applesauce, and toast. Here's a low-fat version of everyone's favorite Southern pudding, guaranteed to delight as long as you keep the "tofu" word to yourself. Be sure to make the dessert at least 8 hours and preferably a day in advance so the ingredients have time to soften and mellow.

3 tablespoons cornstarch

$^1/_3$ cup plus 2 tablespoons demerara or
    turbinado sugar

3 cups organic reduced-fat (2%) milk

3 egg yolks

2 teaspoons vanilla extract

40 reduced-fat Nilla Wafers (about half an
    11-ounce box)

$3^1/_2$ bananas, fully ripe but not brown, sliced

In a heavy saucepan, combine the cornstarch and sugar. Whisk in the milk until blended. Cook over medium heat, whisking often, for about 5 minutes, until the milk comes to a boil and thickens. Reduce the heat to medium-low and simmer for 2 minutes. Remove from the heat.

In a small bowl, beat the egg yolks lightly. Gradually whisk in about ¾ cup of the hot milk to warm them. Whisk the egg yolks into the remaining milk in the pan. Cook over medium heat, whisking, for 1 minute. Remove from the heat, scrape the custard into a bowl, and let cool to tepid. Whisk in the vanilla.

Reserve 2 of the cookies for garnish and break up the rest. Arrange a thin layer of the broken cookies in the bottom of a 1½- to 2-quart baking dish or soufflé dish. Cover with 1 sliced banana and about 1 cup of the vanilla custard. Repeat these layers 2 more times, using all the custard at the end. Cover and refrigerate overnight.

Shortly before serving, coarsely crush the 2 cookies. Decorate the pudding with the remaining banana slices and crushed cookies.

# Peach and Blackberry Crisp

Serves 4 to 6

When fruit is in season, it offers a fine way to indulge in dessert without excess sugar, which can lead to heartburn. The riper and sweeter the fruit, the less sugar you'll need. While *cobbler* is a pretty word, it involves a lot of dough and a good bit of butter, which isn't easy to digest. This *crisp* offers a delightful low-fat topping studded with nuts and oats. Serve plain, with a drizzle of heavy cream, or with a small scoop of low-fat frozen yogurt.

4 large ripe peaches, preferably organic

1 pint blackberries

$1/3$ cup plus 2 tablespoons unbleached all-purpose flour

$1/4$ cup plus 3 tablespoons light brown sugar

1 teaspoon cinnamon

$1/4$ teaspoon ground cardamom

$1/3$ cup rolled oats

2 tablespoons unsalted butter, cut into small dice

1 tablespoon sunflower oil

3 tablespoons coarsely chopped pecans

Heavy cream or low-fat frozen yogurt, for topping (optional)

Preheat the oven to 350°F.

If the peaches are not organic, peel them by dropping them into a pot of boiling water for about 10 seconds. Remove and rinse under cold running water. The peels should slip right off. Cut the peaches in half and remove the pits, then cut into $1/2$-inch slices.

In a $1^1/2$- to 2-quart baking dish, toss the sliced peaches and the blackberries with 2 tablespoons of the flour, 3 tablespoons of the brown sugar, $1/2$ teaspoon of the cinnamon, and the cardamom.

In small bowl, combine the remaining $1/3$ cup flour, $1/4$ cup brown sugar, and $1/2$ teaspoon cinnamon with the rolled oats. Toss to mix. Add the butter and toss to coat the cubes with the dry ingredients. Drizzle on the oil. Pinch the mixture between your fingertips until it is evenly blended and has the texture of coarse meal. Mix the pecans into the topping.

Pick up small bits of the topping and squeeze in your hand so it sticks together; then crumble over the fruit in the baking dish. Repeat until you use all the topping. Leave some larger chunks as well as some looser bits of topping.

Bake the crisp for 25 to 30 minutes, until the fruit is bubbling and the topping is very lightly browned. Serve warm or at room temperature either plain or with the topping of your choice.

# Blueberry-Mango Parfaits

## Serves 4

Fruit and nuts are both great sources of fiber as well as vitamins and antioxidants. And they complement each other beautifully. Yogurt is considered a probiotic. That means it contains live organisms—so-called good bacteria—that aid digestion. To keep this a lean treat, use a low-fat Greek-style yogurt, or drain plain goat's milk yogurt in a coffee filter for an hour or two. If you halve the sugar, omit the vanilla, and add some toasted rolled oats, this makes a lovely breakfast treat.

2/3 cup pecan halves or pieces

2 ripe mangoes, preferably yellow Ataulfo

1 pint blueberries

2 1/2 tablespoons demerara or turbinado sugar

1/2 teaspoon ground cinnamon

1 cup plain low-fat Greek-style yogurt or drained
     goat's milk yogurt

2 tablespoons unsweetened shredded coconut

1/2 teaspoon vanilla extract

Preheat the oven to 325°F. Toast the pecans for 5 to 7 minutes, until very lightly browned. Or microwave on a plate for 45 to 60 seconds. Let cool slightly, then chop the nuts very coarsely, leaving some bigger pieces.

Peel the mangoes and slice the flesh off the pit. Cut the mango into about 1/2-inch dice. Toss with the blueberries, 1 tablespoon of the sugar, the cinnamon, and all but 1 1/2 tablespoons of the chopped nuts.

In a small bowl, blend the yogurt with the coconut, the remaining 1 1/2 tablespoons sugar, and the vanilla extract.

Layer the fruit and nut mixture and flavored yogurt in 4 parfait glasses or wine glasses. Sprinkle the remaining 1 1/2 tablespoons toasted pecans on top.

NOTE: If strawberries don't bother your stomach, you can substitute them for the blueberries, or use half and half for really pretty color.

# White Chocolate Mousse with Raspberry Swirl

Serves 6

Light and exceptionally easy, this lovely mousse can be whipped up in minutes. Garnish with a few fresh berries or a sprinkling of pistachios.

Raspberry Sauce (recipe follows)

$1/3$ cup heavy cream

6 ounces white chocolate, chopped, or 1 cup white chocolate bits

$1/2$ pound silken tofu

2 teaspoons vanilla extract

Fresh berries, for garnish

Shelled and roasted pistachio nuts, for garnish

Prepare the sauce and set aside.

In a small heavy saucepan, heat the heavy cream until simmering. Add the white chocolate and remove from the heat. Stir until the white chocolate is melted and the mixture is smooth. Let cool slightly.

In a food processor, combine the tofu and white chocolate cream. Add the vanilla and process for 30 to 60 seconds.

Divide among 6 bowls. Spoon on 1 to 2 tablespoons of the raspberry sauce and use a blunt knife or small offset spatula to swirl through the mousse. Cover and refrigerate for at least 2 hours, until set.

To serve, drizzle a little of the remaining sauce on top, pass on the side, or reserve for another use. Garnish with the berries and pistachios.

## RASPBERRY SAUCE

Makes about $1^1/2$ cups

1 (10-ounce) package frozen raspberries (no sugar added)

2 tablespoons seedless raspberry or marionberry preserves

1 tablespoon demerara or turbinado sugar

In a food processor, whirl together the raspberries, preserves, and sugar until blended and smooth. If you want to remove the seeds, pass through the medium disk of a food mill.

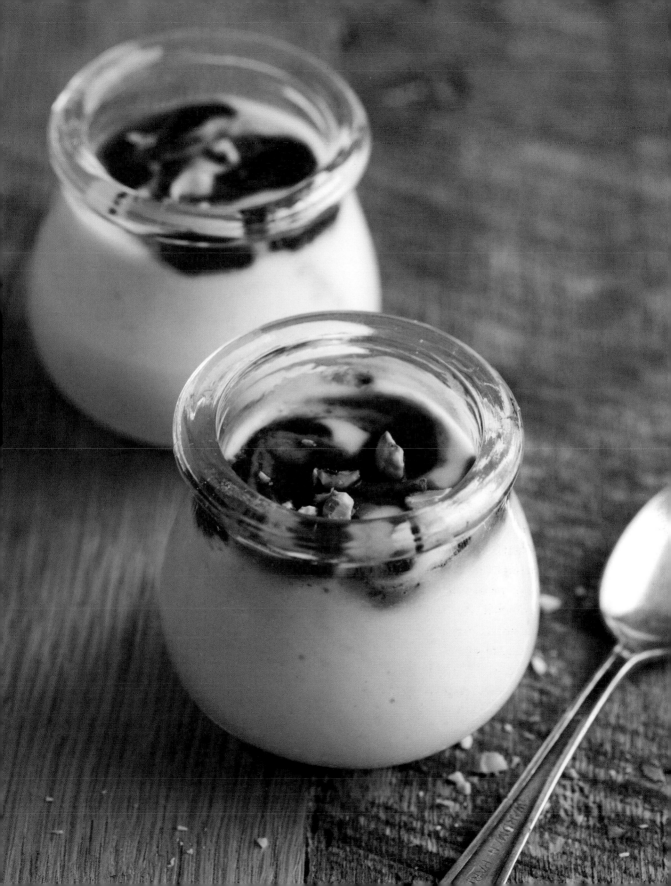

# Coconut Flan
## Serves 8

Everyone loves flan, especially me since my heritage is Cuban. While the custard is rich, it is easily digestible, and the added coconut here makes it even more so. The important thing to remember if you suffer from GERD is that dessert should not be a habit but a treat. And you really do need to leave room for it. If you feel stuffed after dinner, wait an hour or so before dessert. Just make sure your last bite of food still leaves at least three hours before bedtime. If not, skip it and enjoy dessert for breakfast; otherwise, you'll pay the price.

1 cup demerara or turbinado sugar

3 whole eggs

2 egg yolks

1 (14-ounce) can sweetened condensed milk

1 (14-ounce) can unsweetened coconut milk

1 1/2 cups half-and-half

1 1/2 teaspoons vanilla extract

3/4 cup flaked sweetened coconut, toasted
  (see note)

Put the sugar in a small saucepan with 3 or 4 tablespoons water. Slowly bring to a simmer, stirring to dissolve the sugar. Boil over medium heat without stirring at all for 3 to 5 minutes, until the syrup turns a nut-brown color. Remove from the heat and immediately pour into a deep-dish glass pie pan or 2-inch deep round casserole, tilting the pan so the caramel covers the bottom and a little of the sides. (Don't worry; this doesn't have to be perfect.)

Preheat the oven to 325°F. Pour about 3/4 inch of water into a large roasting pan and place it on a rack in the center of the oven.

In a mixing bowl, whisk the eggs and egg yolks to break them up. Whisk in the condensed milk until thoroughly blended. Then add the coconut milk, half-and-half, and vanilla. Blend well. Pour into the caramel-lined pan.

Place the pie dish in the roasting pan in the oven. Bake for 1 hour 15 minutes. Carefully remove the dish from the water bath and set on a rack. Let cool for 10 to 15 minutes. Then place a sheet of plastic wrap directly on the custard and refrigerate until chilled, at least 4 hours or overnight.

To serve, set a large round platter over the pie pan and quickly invert to unmold the flan. The caramel syrup will run down around it. Sprinkle the toasted coconut on top. Cut into 8 wedges, making sure everyone gets a spoonful of caramel syrup, as well.

NOTE: To toast the coconut, preheat the oven to 325°F. Spread out the coconut on a baking sheet and bake for 8 to 10 minutes, until lightly browned. Watch carefully, because sweetened coconut can burn quickly.

# Cocoa Meringues

Makes about 3 dozen; allow 2 per serving

Chocolate is an absolute no-no when it comes to GERD. But a life without chocolate may feel a bit grim. Cocoa retains the flavor but little of the fat. So here are some small bites to enjoy upon occasion. If properly stored, they will keep well for up to 5 days. That's still not long enough to ration these properly; so be sure to share with some favorite friends or make half a batch.

3/4 cup organic cane sugar

1/2 cup egg whites (from about 4 large egg whites)

1/3 cup confectioners' sugar

3 tablespoons unsweetened cocoa powder

Preheat the oven to 300°F. Line 2 cookie sheets with parchment paper.

In a small saucepan, combine the cane sugar with 3 tablespoons water. Cover the pot and bring to a rolling boil over medium-low heat. Remove the lid and boil without stirring until the syrup reaches 238°F (soft ball stage) on a candy thermometer.

While the cane sugar cooks, place the egg whites in the large bowl of an electric mixer. In a small bowl, sift together the confectioners' sugar and cocoa.

When the cane sugar reaches temperature, begin whipping the egg whites on medium speed. Carefully pour the syrup in a thin stream into the whites, avoiding the beaters so the syrup does not splatter; be careful because melted sugar causes nasty burns. Continue to whip the meringue until the whites are stiff. Sift the cocoa mixture over the top of the meringue and gently fold by hand with a rubber spatula until evenly blended.

Scoop the egg whites into a piping bag fitted with a large (1/2-inch) star tip and pipe 1 1/2-inch swirls onto the lined cookie sheets. Or use 2 large spoons to form neat mounds.

Bake the meringues for 1 hour, rotating the trays after 30 minutes. Allow them to cool completely on the baking sheet, then pack them in an airtight container so they remain crisp.

# Pecan Tea Cookies

Makes about 2 dozen; allow 2 or 3 per serving

These crisp little cookies are delightful with herbal tea or as an accompaniment to dress up fruit salad.

1 cup unbleached all-purpose flour, preferably organic

3/4 cup pecan pieces

1/2 teaspoon baking soda

1/3 cup coconut oil

1/2 cup plus 2 tablespoons organic cane sugar

1/2 teaspoon almond extract

1 egg white

Preheat the oven to 350°F. Line 2 cookie sheets with parchment or cover with silicone liners.

In a food processor, pulse together the flour, pecans, and baking soda until they form a coarse meal. Set the dry ingredients aside.

In a separate bowl, whisk together the coconut oil, sugar, and almond extract until blended. Beat in the egg white until well blended. Add the dry ingredients and stir with a wooden spoon until thoroughly mixed.

Drop the dough by heaping teaspoons onto the prepared cookie sheets, leaving about 2 inches in between. Bake for 12 minutes, or until the cookies are just beginning to brown around the edges. Transfer to a wire rack and let cool before eating.

# Very Berry Mousse

Serves 5

Here's an instant dessert that will have you licking the spoon. And that's fine, because each serving contains only 130 calories. Do not—I repeat, DO NOT—tell your friends what the base is. Or, at least, not until they beg you for the recipe. Serve topped with fresh berries, if you like.

8 ounces silken tofu

10 ounces frozen marionberries, raspberries, or strawberries

1/4 cup plus 2 tablespoons demerara or turbinado sugar

1/4 cup heavy cream

1 teaspoon rose water

1/2 teaspoon vanilla extract

Combine all the ingredients in a food processor; no need to thaw the berries. Pulse until the berries are evenly distributed. Then process until smooth.

Divide among 5 dessert dishes. Serve at once or cover and refrigerate for up to 3 hours.

# Rice Pudding with Pistachios and Dried Cherries

## Serves 6 to 8

Soothing and yummy, you'll find this cardamom-scented pudding makes it hard to put down your spoon. Though by now, if you're following the Acid Reflux Solution, you know you must. Nonetheless, rice is easy to digest and using soy milk produces the lightest, leanest pudding possible, allowing a generous portion.

1 cup jasmine or basmati rice

$1/2$ cup reduced-fat coconut milk

$1^3/4$ cups enriched organic soy milk (see note)

$1/3$ cup demerara or turbinado sugar

$3/8$ teaspoon ground cardamom

$1/3$ cup dried cherries

$1/3$ cup chopped, shelled, and roasted pistachio nuts

In a 2- to $2^1/2$-quart heavy saucepan, bring $3^1/2$ cups water to a boil. Add the rice and boil for 10 minutes. Remove from the heat, cover, and let stand for 5 minutes. Drain off any excess water.

Return the rice to the pan and add the coconut milk, $1^1/2$ cups of the soy milk, the sugar, and cardamom. Bring to a simmer, reduce the heat to low, and cook, uncovered, for about 10 minutes, until the pudding thickens.

Add the cherries and all but $1^1/2$ tablespoons of the nuts. Stir in the remaining $1/4$ cup soy milk and let stand for at least 5 minutes. Serve the rice pudding warm, at room temperature, or slightly chilled, with the remaining pistachios sprinkled on top.

NOTE: For best flavor, choose a neutral soy milk that does not have added sugar or vanilla flavoring, such as organic Eden brand.

# MEDICAL TECHNOLOGY TO THE RESCUE

**BY NOW, I HOPE YOU UNDERSTAND** how an appropriate diet and the very reasonable lifestyle adaptations we've detailed can begin the healing process and, for all practical purposes, eventually eliminate acid reflux from your life. Maybe you've even started some of my easy recommendations for alleviating GERD. We've also gone over what causes reflux and what kinds of medications can help. But some people—perhaps a small minority, but an important minority if you are one of them—have an intractable problem. That is, no matter what they do, their symptoms persist.

Sometimes acid reflux cannot be alleviated if too much damage has already occurred before remedial diet and lifestyle changes were adopted. Over time, repeated bouts of reflux may have caused permanent scarring and other complications. Or there could be a genetic or structural physiological reason why some people do not respond to palliative measures.

After diligently making healthy lifestyle changes and following the Acid Reflux Solution for several months, if your symptoms still don't improve, the first thing that must be done is to stop guessing what is going on.

Long-term complications of GERD can be serious and should not be left to assumptions. I already advised you to consult your doctor at the outset to make sure your symptoms were, indeed, simply the result of heartburn and not angina or another medical problem. Your doctor may have approved the over-the-counter medications you were taking, making sure they did not interact with any other prescriptions you were on, or prescribed a stronger antacid for temporary use if it was absolutely necessary in the short term while you continued to manage your symptoms naturally.

If after three months, despite everything you try, painful reflux not only flares up intermittently but persists on a regular basis, I strongly encourage you to return to your physician to put a halt to the progression of the disease. Don't take this as an ominous warning and whatever you do, don't panic. It simply means that something further may need to be done. We experts in the field have many tools in our kit.

What's likely to happen when you consult a physician at this stage? A doctor's job is to review symptoms, analyzing them within the context of both the individual patient and extensive clinical experience with thousands of patients, and come up with an answer, or diagnosis. But without testing or seeing with his or her own eyes what's going on, even an educated assumption is still a guess. With gastrointestinal issues, when chronic symptoms won't quit, we doctors think it's important to take a literal look inside the upper gastrointestinal (GI) tract—what I like to call "introspection."

## Endoscopy

So first of all, there's a good chance your doctor will want to take a peek inside your body to see what's actually going on. Since none of us is Superman or Superwoman, X-ray vision won't do it, but an endoscope will. What is essentially a very sophisticated system of fiber optics allows us to see why some people's symptoms are not going away or have progressed to a more serious state. Sometimes an endoscopy can help prove how serious your GERD is. If you have tried our recommendations and nothing has helped, perhaps laparoscopic repair of your LES is the only alternative. In order to prove this, endoscopy combined with monitoring of the pH level is needed first.

The endoscope is a long, thin, flexible tube with a microchip on its tip that transmits real-time color images of the inside of your body to many screens within the procedure room. It's much the same as a video camera only it's the size of the head of a pin. We thread this tool down into the esophagus, sometimes going all the way to the stomach or even to the duodenum (the beginning of the small intestines), to get a good look. While endoscopy is a simple procedure, trust me, it's a little like flying a plane; you can't just pick up the controls and go. It takes a GI specialist like me two to three years to learn how to maneuver an endoscope properly and use it to best advantage. So you don't need to worry, because anyone performing an endoscopy has years of training and experience under his or her belt. If your doctor says you need to have an endoscopy, know that it is a safe and effective way of treating many complications of GERD.

An endoscope allows us not just to look inside but also to fix things there. Specifically, we can perform microsurgeries by inserting small instruments into the endoscope, which allows us to take biopsies, stop bleedings, inject medications, and use suction to attach tiny pH monitors onto the surface of the esophagus. It's these monitors that tell us when a patient is experiencing reflux and how high the acid is traveling.

In order to have an endoscopy performed, you must first be put into a deep sleep—what we call "twilight sleep." It is not general anesthesia as in a surgery, but a very deep amnestic sleep. Technically, you are not unconscious, but you will not remember a thing about the procedure afterward, so it feels as if you have been put under. This is a very safe and highly monitored part of the procedure. All you

## Gastroparesis

As mentioned, some conditions that mimic GERD are caused by other factors. One of them is gastroparesis, or an abnormally slow emptying of the stomach after eating. This can lead to feeling bloated or nauseated, which often happens with GERD, but can also be a consequence of diabetes. Now, don't get scared. I'm not saying that heartburn is a symptom of diabetes or that it leads to diabetes. I'm saying that if you have a diagnosis of diabetes, that may be an underlying reason for the reflux. For unknown reasons, uncontrolled blood sugar—maybe from before diagnosis or if there are challenges in keeping glucose levels within the prescribed limits—can damage the vagus nerve. This is the major nerve that automatically regulates a number of functions, including digestion, in ways you don't even feel.

It's important to know whether this is the cause of your problem, because there are other medical measures and medications that can help. Some of the lifestyle recommendations I make in the next chapter for treating GERD, such as eating smaller meals and remaining upright for at least an hour after a meal, may help alleviate symptoms. You also want to make sure your food is soft and moist, which may make it pass through more easily. And losing weight, even just 5 percent of your body mass, and maintaining blood glucose levels between 80 and 120, will likely help. If they don't or if symptoms return, your doctor may want to prescribe a drug to stimulate the vagus nerve and increase what we doctors call "gastric motility," the movement of food through the gastrointestinal, or GI, tract.

remember is going to sleep and waking up. In the meantime, your upper intestinal tract has been thoroughly examined and the problem at hand hopefully resolved.

The acid in the esophagus can be measured by having the endoscope suction a very small pH monitor to the wall of the esophagus. For 48 hours after waking up, this high-tech device sends information to a receiver the patient wears on his or her belt. It shows every single occurrence of reflux, detailing when it occurred, how long it lasted, how much acid came up, and so on. A complicated scoring system tells us how bad the reflux is. A high result is almost always enough reason to have surgical correction for GERD.

## Long-Term Complications

The reason it's so important to obtain this material proof of disease is that some of the physiological conditions associated with GERD and long-term complications can be dangerous. Among the most common are:

- Esophagitis
- Barrett's esophagus
- Strictures of the esophagus

Esophagitis is a chronic, painful inflammation of the esophagus caused by long-term repeated acid reflux. Sure, we sometimes treat symptoms that are suggestive of esophagitis after a simple office visit, but if those symptoms don't improve, an endoscopy is a must. The only way of truly confirming a diagnosis of esophagitis is by looking inside to see the tearing away of the esophageal lining caused by caustic stomach acid.

One reason esophagitis concerns us, besides the obvious discomfort to the patient, is that if it continues, the reflux can eventually lead to what is called "Barrett's esophagus," a dangerous condition that shows changes in the tissue that lines the esophagus. The cells morph into an abnormal precancerous state, meaning that they are not currently growing out of control, but they possess the possibility of doing so. Recently developed procedures allow us to use the endoscope to freeze or dissolve away these spots of abnormal tissue from the lining of the esophagus, just as you might have a precancerous lesion removed from your arm. Some follow-up endoscopies are required, much like a dermatologist would monitor the site where a cancerous mole was removed, but the fact that there is now a potential cure for Barrett's esophagus is heartening.

Another complication of long-term esophagitis is the development of esophageal strictures, or closures. Every time stomach acid burns the esophagus, it can leave behind a scar. It is no wonder that years of scarring can cause a narrowing of the esophagus, to the point where food cannot pass through. If you have ever eaten a piece of juicy steak, swallowed, and had the meat caught in your chest, then you know what I am talking about. It is terrifying! Not even saliva can pass through. What makes it an emergency is that no food or water will pass unless this blockage is cleared. In this case, we really do have to clean out the pipe.

Esophageal strictures constitute a true medical emergency. In this instance, an endoscopy is crucial not only to remove the food that is stuck but also to open up the passage so it doesn't happen again. Much like an angioplasty in a clogged artery, we use the endoscope to pass an inflated balloon through the esophagus, pushing the scar tissue back and permanently stretching and tearing the stricture so that food will no longer get caught. Unless, of course, GERD continues, in which case a more permanent, surgical solution may be needed.

## Surgery

Surgeries to correct complications from intractable GERD are no longer the arduous procedures they were in the "olden days," when working on the esophagus was as complicated as open-heart surgery. Nowadays, medical science is much more sophisticated, and most surgical techniques are laparoscopic and minimally invasive. We make three small incisions in the abdomen to reach the area we need to work on and insert three thin tubes. One inflates the belly so there is room to work, another holds the camera so the doctor can see what he's doing, and the third is a tiny robotic arm that manipulates the surgical tools.

The most common of these laparoscopic operations to correct problems of acid reflux is the "Nissen fundoplication." In the simplest of terms, this operation tightens the LES by literally stitching it up using the fiberoptic tools I've described to you. Usually measurements of the LES tone are done during surgery to make sure the LES is not tightened too much. This procedure is safe, effective, and long lasting in its effectiveness. It can be performed on an outpatient basis but usually requires a day of hospital observation.

Surgery for treatment of GERD or its complications should always be the last resort. Be sure to educate yourself on what your physician is recommending and don't be shy about asking questions until you are satisfied that this is the correct solution for you. But if no other measures work, do not hesitate to go ahead with the procedure to prevent progression of the disease, though I do encourage you to choose a surgeon who has done many of these operations.

As for us, well, we are trying to help anyone who can avoid the need for surgery just as we are trying to help you avoid unnecessary medication. They are both appropriate solutions, at the correct time, but only if nothing else works. Lifestyle modifications come first. I hope I have convinced you that you can control GERD in a much more permanent and healthy way with diet. You don't have to starve yourself or sacrifice. But you do have to be conscious and aware of what and how you eat. In the long run, this will serve you very well, not just to control GERD but also to make you healthier all around. So try the recipes, and enjoy *The Acid Reflux Solution* as much as we enjoyed creating it.

# BIBLIOGRAPHY

Anvari M., C. Allen, J. Marshall, D. Armstrong, R. Goeree, W. Ungar, and C. Goldsmith. "A Randomized Controlled Trial of Laparoscopic Nissen Fundoplication Versus Proton Pump Inhibitors for the Treatment of Patients with Chronic Gastroesophageal Reflux Disease (GERD): 3-Year Outcomes." *Surgical Endoscopy* 25, no. 8 (2011): 2547–54.

Ayazi S., J. A. Hagan, L. S. Chan et al. "Obesity and Gastroesophageal Reflux: Quantifying the Association between Body Mass Index, Esophageal Acid Exposure, and Lower Esophageal Sphincter Status in a Large Series of Patients with Reflux Symptoms." *Journal of Gastrointestinal Surgery* 13, no. 8 (August 2009): 1440–47.

Baldi F., C. Cavoli, R. Solimando et al. "Reflux Oesophagitis in Italy (Diomede Project)." *Digestive and Liver Disease* 40, no. 6 (2008): 405–11.

Berkson, D. L. *Healthy Digestion the Natural Way.* Wiley, 2000.

Bernstein, M., and A. S. Luggen. *Nutrition for the Older Adult.* Jones and Bartlett, 2010.

Blondeau K., V. Boecxstaens, L. Van Oudenhove et al. "Increasing Body Weight Enhances Prevalence and Proximal Extent of Reflux in GERD Patients 'On' and 'Off' PPI Therapy." *Neurogastroenterology & Motility* 23, no. 8 (2011): 724–27.

Brown, J. E. *Nutrition through the Life Cycle*, 3rd ed. Thomson Wadsworth, 2010.

Daley, C., A. Abbott, P. A. Doyle, G. A. Nader, and S. Larson. "A Review of Fatty Acid Profiles and Antioxidant Content in Grass-Fed and Grain-Fed Beef." *Nutrition Journal* 10, no. 9 (March 2010): 10.

De Groot, N., J. S. Burgerhart, P. C. Van De Meebertg et al. "Systematic Review: The Effects of Conservative and Surgical Treatment for Obesity on Gastro-Oesophageal Reflux Disease." *Alimentary Pharmacology & Therapeutics* 30, no. 11–12 (December 2009): 1091–1102.

Festi, D., E. Scaioli, F. Baldi et al. "Body Weight, Lifestyle, Dietary Habits and Gastroesophageal Reflux Disease." *World Journal of Gastroenterology* 15, no. 14 (April 2009): 1690–1701.

Fisher, B. L., A. Pennathur, J. L. Mutnick, and A. G. Little. "Obesity Correlates with Gastroesophageal Reflux." *Digestive Diseases and Sciences* 44, no. 11 (November 1999): 2290–94.

Fock, K. M., and C. H. Poh. "Gastroesophageal Reflux Disease." *Journal of Gastroenterology* 45, no. 8 (2010): 808–15.

Friedenberg, F. K., M. Xanthopoulos, G. D. Foster, and J. E. Richter. "The Association between Gastroesophageal Reflux Disease and Obesity." *The American Journal of Gastroenterology* 103, no. 8 (August 2008): 2111–22.

Gonlachanvit, S. "Are Rice and Spicy Diet Good for Functional Gastrointestinal Disorders?" *Journal of Neurogastroenterology & Motility* 2 (April 2010): 1331–38.

Hampel, H. "Meta-Analysis: Obesity and the Risk for Gastroesophageal Reflux Disease and Its Complications." *Annals of Internal Medicine* 143, no. 3 (2005): 199–211.

Heine, R. G. "Gastroesophageal Reflux Disease, Colic and Constipation in Infants with Food Allergy." *Current Opinion in Allergy and Clinical Immunology* 6, no. 3 (June 2006): 220–25.

IMS Institute for Healthcare Informatics. *The Use of Medicines in the United States: Review of 2010.* IMS Institute for Healthcare Informatics, 2011.

Katz, L. C., R. Just, and D. O. Castell. "Body Position Affects Recumbent Postprandial Reflux." *Journal of Clinical Gastroenterology* 4 (June 1994): 280–83.

Kubo, A., G. Block, C. P. Quesenberry, P. Buffler, and D. A. Corley. "Effects of Dietary Fiber, Fats, and Meat Intakes on the Risk of Barrett's Esophagus." *Nutrition and Cancer* 61, no. 5 (2009): 607–16.

Lien, H., C. C. Wang, J. Y. Hsu et al. "Classical Reflux Symptoms, Hiatus Hernia and Overweight Independently Predict Pharyngeal Acid Exposure in Patients with Suspected Reflux Laryngitis." *Alimentary Pharmacology and Therapeutics* 33, no. 1 (2010): 89–98.

Lipski, E. *Digestive Wellness.* McGraw-Hill, 2005.

Lodato F., F. Azzaroli, L. Turco, N. Mazzella et al. "Adverse Effects of Proton Pump Inhibitors." *Best Practice & Research Clinical Gastroenterology* 24, no. 2 (April 2010): 193–201.

Lukić, M., A. Segec, I. Segeca et al. "The Role of Nutrition in the Pathogenesis of Gastroesophageal Reflux Disease, Barrett's Oesophagus and Oesophageal Adenocarcinoma." *Collegium Antropologicum* 34, no. 3 (September 2010): 905–9.

Magee, Elaine. *Tell Me What to Eat If I Have Acid Reflux.* New Page Books, 2009.

Mahan, L. K., and S. Escott-Stump. *Krause's Food & Nutrition Therapy*, 12th ed. Elsevier, Inc., 2008.

Meining, A., and M. Classen. "The Role of Diet and Lifestyle Measures in the Pathogenesis and Treatment of Gastroesophageal Reflux Disease." *The American Journal of Gastroenterology* 95, no. 10 (October 2000): 2692–97.

Merwat, S. N., and S. J. Spechler. "Might the Use of Acid-Suppresssive Medications Predispose to the Development of Eosinophilic Esophagitis?" *The American Journal of Gastroenterology* 104, no. 8 (2009): 1897–1902.

Murao T., K. Sakurai, S. Jihara et al. "Lifestyle Change Influences on GERD in Japan: A Study of Participants in a Health Examination Program." *Digestive Diseases and Sciences* (April 13, 2011).

Murphy, D. W., and D. O. Castell. "Chocolate and Heartburn: Evidence of Increased Esophageal Acid Exposure after Chocolate Ingestion." *The American Journal of Gastroenterology* 83, no. 6 (June 1988): 633–36.

Murray, L., B. Johnston, L. Athene, I. Harvey et al. "Relationship between Body Mass and Gastro-Oesophageal Reflux Symptoms: The Bristol Helicobacter Project." *International Journal of Epidemiology* 32 (2003): 645–50.

Nachman, F., H. Vázquez., A. Gonzalez et al. "Gastroesophageal Reflux Symptoms in Patients with Celiac Disease and the Effects of a Gluten-Free Diet." *Clinical Gastroenterology and Hepatology* 9, no. 3 (2010): 214–19.

Nebel, O. T., M. F. Fornes , and D. O. Castell . "Symptomatic Gastroesophageal Reflux: Incidence and Precipitating Factors." *The American Journal of Digestive Diseases* 21, no. 11 (November 1976): 953–56.

Nilsson, M., R. Johnsen, W. Ye et al. "Lifestyle Related Risk Factors in the Aetiology of Gastro-Esophageal Reflux." *Gut* 53, no. 12 (2004): 1730–35.

Pronsky, Z. M. *Food-Medication Interactions*, 15th ed. Food-Medications Interactions, 2008.

Rogers, M. D., and A. Sherry. *No More Heartburn: Stop the Pain in 30 Days—Naturally!* Kensington Books, 2000.

Sakamoto, Y., M. Inamori, T. Iwasaki et al. "Relationship between Upper Gastrointestinal Symptoms and Diet Therapy: Examination Using Frequency Scale for the Symptoms of Gastroesophageal Reflux Disease." *Hepato-Gastroenterology* 57, no. 104 (November-December 2010): 1635–38.

Sklar, J., and A. Cohen. *Eating for Acid Reflux: A Handbook and Cookbook for Those with Heartburn*. Da Capo Press, 2003.

Souza, R. F. "Bringing GERD Management Up to PAR-2." *The American Journal of Gastroenterology* 105, no. 9 (September 2010): 1944–46.

Spergel, J. M., T. Andrews, T. F. Brown-Whitehorn et al. "Treatment of Eosinophilic Esophagitis with Specific Food Elimination Diet Directed by a Combination of Skin Prick and Patch Tests." *Annals of Allergy, Asthma and Immunology* 95, no. 4 (2005): 336–43.

Stephanidis, D. et al. "Guidelines for Surgical Treatment of Gastroesophageal Reflux Disease." *Society of American and Gastrointestinal and Endoscopic Surgeons*, 2010: http://www.sages.org/publication/id/22.

Tsai, M., H. L. Lin, C. C. Lin et al. "Increased Risk of Concurrent Asthma among Patients with Gastroesophageal Reflux Disease: A Nationwide Population-Based Study." *European Journal of Gastroenterology & Hepatology* 10 (2010): 1169–73.

Usai, P., R. Manca, R. Cuomo, M. A. Lai, L. Russo, and M. F. Boi. "Effect of Gluten-Free Diet on Preventing Recurrence of Gastroesophageal Reflux Disease-Related Symptoms in Adult Celiac Patients with Nonerosive Reflux Disease." *Journal of Gastroenterology and Hepatology* 9 (2009): 1368–72.

Vemulapalli, R. "Diet and Lifestyle Modifications in the Management of Gastroesophageal Reflux Disease." *Nutrition in Clinical Practice* 23, no. 3 (2008): 193–98.

Wendland, B. E., and L. M. Ruffolo. *Chronic Heartburn: Managing Acid Reflux and GERD through Understanding, Diet and Lifestyle*. Robert Rose, 2006.

Yoshikawa, I., M. Nagato, M. Yamasaki, K. Kume, and M. Otsuki. "Long-Term Treatment with Proton Pump Inhibitor Is Associated with Undesired Weight Gain." *World Journal of Gastroenterology* 15, no. 38 (2009): 1494–98.

# ABOUT THE AUTHORS

**JORGE E. RODRIGUEZ, MD**, is a board-certified internist and gastroenterologist who received his medical degree from the University of Miami. He completed his residency in internal medicine at Tulane Medical School in New Orleans, and his fellowship in gastroenterology at Baylor University Medical Center in Dallas. Dr. Rodriguez has established himself as a leader in HIV treatment and intestinal diseases. He has appeared as an expert medical commentator on *CNN News*, *Good Morning America Health*, *The Doctors*, and *The View*. He is an MDVIP-affiliated physician and has had an internal medicine practice in Newport Beach, California, since 1988.

**SUSAN WYLER, MPH, RD**, is a registered dietitian who worked for many years as a cookbook author and food editor, most notably at *Food & Wine* magazine. Her books include *Cooking from a Country Farmhouse*, *Cooking for a Crowd*, and *The Swiss Secret to Optimal Health*, written with Dr. Thomas Rau. Wyler recently graduated from the University of North Carolina at Chapel Hill with a master's degree in public health. She also did advanced field work at the prestigious cancer research hospital Institut de Cancérologie Gustave Roussy in France. She lives in Chapel Hill, North Carolina.

# MEASUREMENT CONVERSION CHARTS

| VOLUME | | |
|---|---|---|
| U.S. | Imperial | Metric |
| 1 tablespoon | $1/2$ fl oz | 15 ml |
| 2 tablespoons | 1 fl oz | 30 ml |
| $1/4$ cup | 2 fl oz | 60 ml |
| $1/3$ cup | 3 fl oz | 90 ml |
| $1/2$ cup | 4 fl oz | 120 ml |
| $2/3$ cup | 5 fl oz ($1/4$ pint) | 150 ml |
| $3/4$ cup | 6 fl oz | 180 ml |
| 1 cup | 8 fl oz ($1/3$ pint) | 240 ml |
| $1^1/4$ cups | 10 fl oz ($1/2$ pint) | 300 ml |
| 2 cups (1 pint) | 16 fl oz ($2/3$ pint) | 480 ml |
| $2^1/2$ cups | 20 fl oz (1 pint) | 600 ml |
| 1 quart | 32 fl oz ($1^2/3$ pint) | 1 l |

| TEMPERATURE | |
|---|---|
| Fahrenheit | Celsius/Gas Mark |
| 250°F | 120°C/gas mark 1/2 |
| 275°F | 135°C/gas mark 1 |
| 300°F | 150°C/gas mark 2 |
| 325°F | 160°C/gas mark 3 |
| 350°F | 180 or 175°C/gas mark 4 |
| 375°F | 190°C/gas mark 5 |
| 400°F | 200°C/gas mark 6 |
| 425°F | 220°C/gas mark 7 |
| 450°F | 230°C/gas mark 8 |
| 475°F | 245°C/gas mark 9 |
| 500°F | 260°C |

| LENGTH | |
|---|---|
| Inch | Metric |
| $1/4$ inch | 6 mm |
| $1/2$ inch | 1.25 cm |
| $3/4$ inch | 2 cm |
| 1 inch | 2.5 cm |
| 6 inches ($1/2$ foot) | 15 cm |
| 12 inches (1 foot) | 30 cm |

| WEIGHT | |
|---|---|
| U.S./Imperial | Metric |
| $1/2$ oz | 15 g |
| 1 oz | 30 g |
| 2 oz | 60 g |
| $1/4$ lb | 115 g |
| $1/3$ lb | 150 g |
| $1/2$ lb | 225 g |
| $3/4$ lb | 350 g |
| 1 lb | 450 g |

# INDEX

**W**

walking, 27, 29, 41–42, 45

walnuts

    Arugula and Hearts of Palm Salad, 94

    Tarragon Chicken Salad with Dried Cherries, Walnuts, and Grapes, 106

    toasting, 94, 106

water, 40–41

Watercress and Cauliflower Soup, 84

Watermelon and Yellow Tomato Salad, 126

weight loss

    benefits of, 31, 57

    effortless, 54–55

    as manifestation of GERD, 10, 16, 57

wheat

    allergies to, 50

    germ, 42

    gluten in, 49

    whole vs. refined, 44

Whipped Cauliflower with Parmesan Cheese, 168

White Chocolate Mousse with Raspberry Swirl, 188

**Y**

yogurt, 187

**Z**

Zantac, 18

zucchini

    Barigoule of Spring Vegetables with Fillet of Flounder, 117

    Black Bean and Grilled Vegetable Chili, 160

    Penne with Zucchini and Mushrooms, 154–55

    Ratatouille with Grilled Eggplant, 169

Published in the United States by Ten Speed Press, an imprint of the Crown Publishing Group, a division of Random House, Inc., New York.
www.crownpublishing.com
www.tenspeed.com

Ten Speed Press and the Ten Speed Press colophon are registered trademarks of Random House, Inc.

Library of Congress Cataloging-in-Publication Data
Rodriguez, Jorge E.
    The acid reflux solution : a cookbook and lifestyle guide for healing heartburn naturally / Jorge E. Rodriguez, Susan Wyler.
        p. cm.
    Includes bibliographical references and index.
1. Gastroesophageal reflux—Popular works. 2. Gastroesophageal reflux—Diet therapy—Recipes. I. Wyler, Susan. II. Title.
    RC815.7R59 2012
    616.3'240654—dc23
        2011033896

ISBN 978-1-60774-227-2
eISBN 978-1-60774-228-9

Printed in China

Design by Katy Brown
Food styling by Karen Shinto
Prop styling by Dani Fisher
Food styling and photography assistance by Victoria Woollard, Jeffrey Larsen, and Irene Chan

10 9 8 7 6 5 4 3

First Edition